THE
MEN'S MAINTENANCE MANUAL

First published 1997 by
Pan Books, an imprint of
Macmillan Publishers Ltd,
25 Eccleston Place,
London SW1W 9NF
and Basingstoke

Associated companies
throughout the world

ISBN 0 330 35376 4

9 8 7 6 5 4 3 2 1

A CIP catalogue entry for this
book is available from the British
Library

All design and photography by
Robin Rout/Photograft, London

Printed by Bath Press
Colour Books, Glasgow

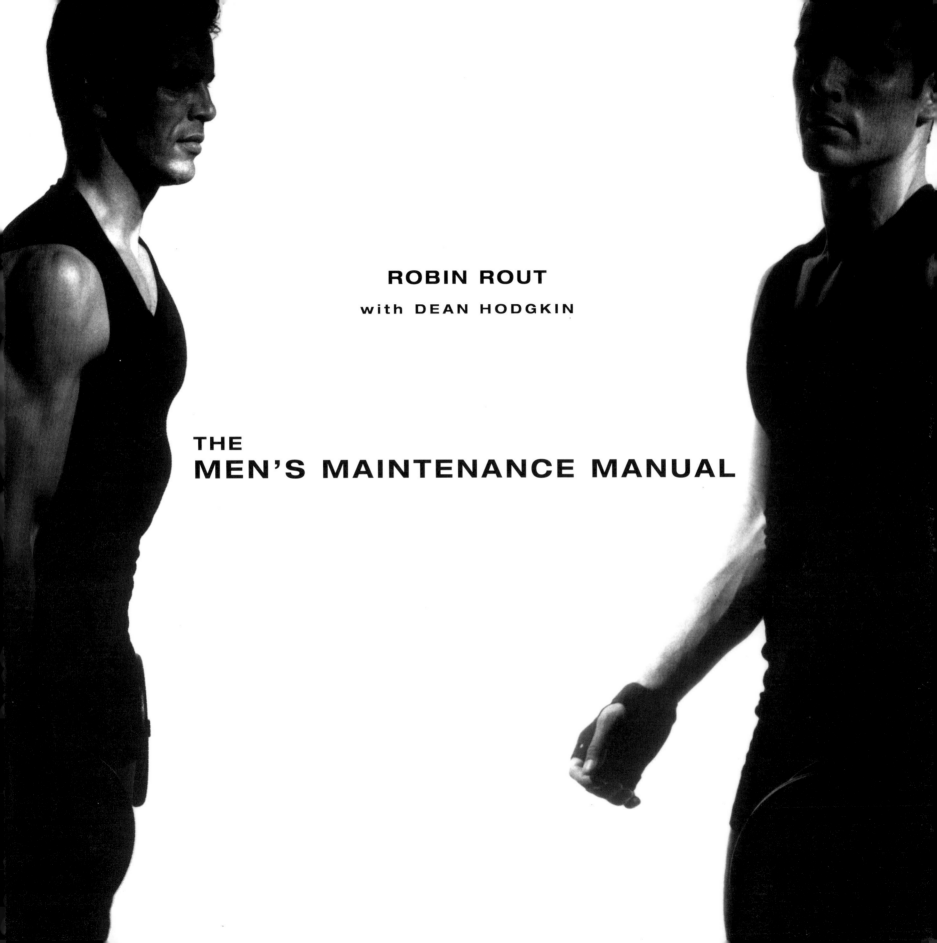

ROBIN ROUT

with DEAN HODGKIN

THE
MEN'S MAINTENANCE MANUAL

This book arose out of a desire to find out how a body that is not in such great shape can get to be that way. If you've already looked along the shelves of your local bookshop you can see that unless you want to be a champion bodybuilder or become a marine commando there is very little to enlighten you on simple gym technique. This book is designed to change this situation. And since most men are squeamish about such a personal matter as the way they look, the body is here referred to as the machine it is; the analogy to cars is not accidental.

CONTENTS

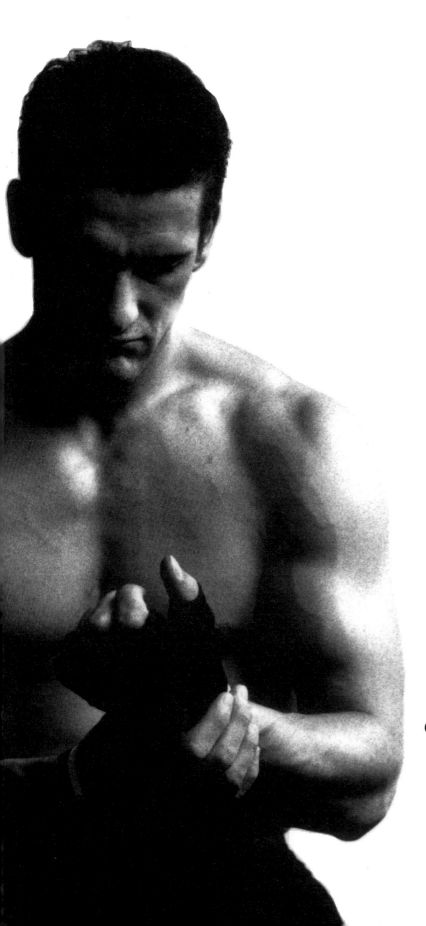

Any word or term underlined in the text is explained in the glossary

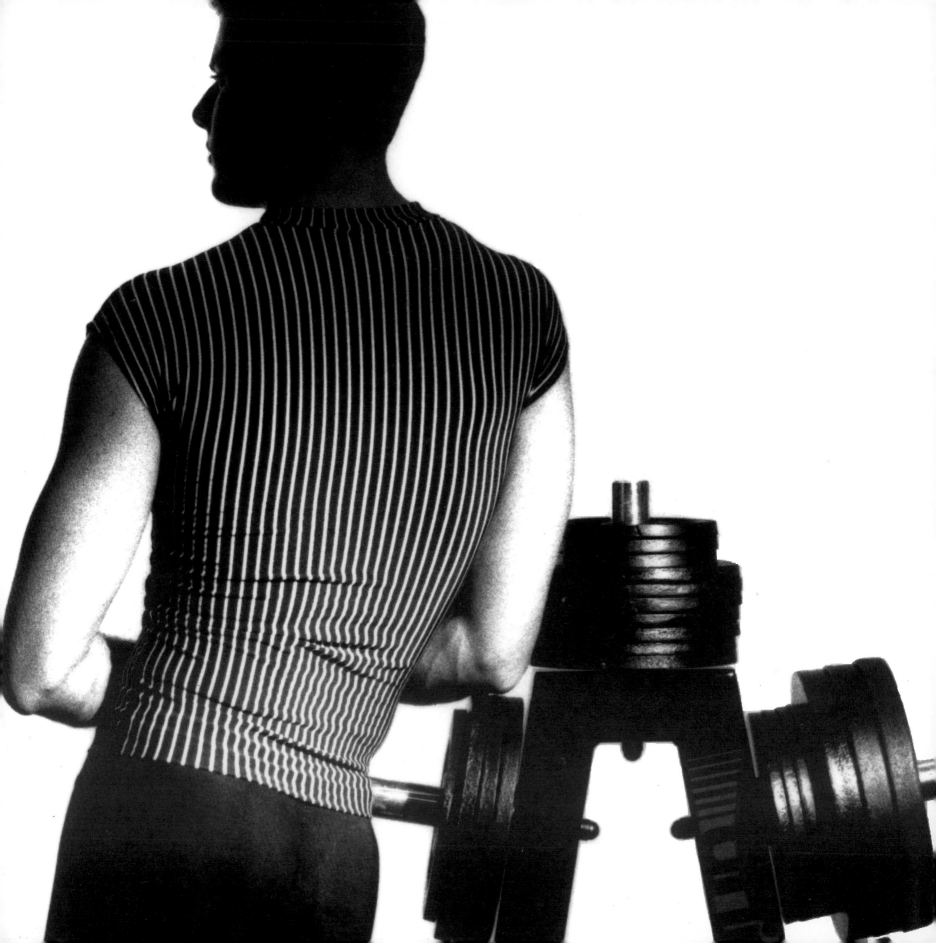

The first time you enter a gym can be a very daunting moment – but then so can entering a garage. A little common sense and basic information will get you going – and this section is designed to help.

IN THE WORKSHOP

Take the time to read through this short section, then get your gym bag and get in there!

HEALTH & SAFETY

Third party damage

Don't let anyone fool you into thinking that a gym is less dangerous than a car workshop. Heavy weights (which can often be moving at speed) are best not involved in collisions of any kind with the human body.

Never forget that when you are working out you are just as much in control of the equivalent of a vehicle on the road – and just as potentially dangerous to yourself and others.

A barbell loaded with 20 kilogram weights in chest press position (see page 34) falling on to your chest without support would be like a low impact head-on collision with a car for a pedestrian.

Gyms, like roads, can become very crowded, particularly at peak times. A popular time for working out is after work in the late afternoon and early evening, so exercise particular caution then to avoid being involved in accidents.

As someone new to the gym you might deliberately choose a time when there are less people around whilst you get the hang of it.

It is also all too easy to switch to cruise control when working out. Any routine can become automatic, so make sure that you always know what is going on around you.

Vehicle inspection

No-one would dream of taking a car out on the road without knowing that it was roadworthy.

It would be foolhardy to do the same with your own body – yet many people do it in relation to exercise without a second thought.

Exertion and stress are integral to any type of exercise and weight training in the gym is one of the most concentrated types of exercise you can undertake.

Be sure that your bill of health is clean by visiting your doctor and explaining they type of exercise you are about to embark on. If you find that your local GP is too busy to see you, ask at the gym that you are considering joining.

Most good gyms retain medically-qualified experts as consultants, and the likelihood is that any of these could easily perform a full medical.

A private consultation may involve you in some cost, but it will be well worth it for the peace of mind it affords you.

It is particularly important to disclose all aspects of your medical history, and relate any family background that is relevant.

Once in the gym, a useful watchword is 'Train – don't strain' to avoid over-ambitious activity which might cause injury.

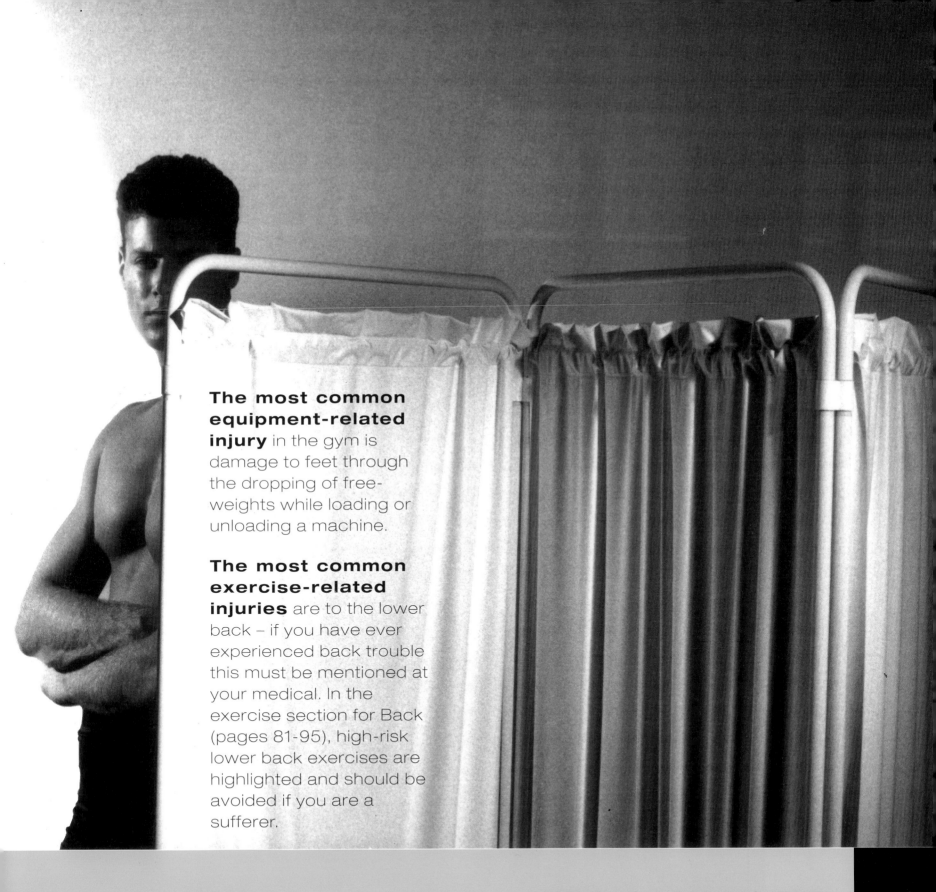

The most common equipment-related injury in the gym is damage to feet through the dropping of free-weights while loading or unloading a machine.

The most common exercise-related injuries are to the lower back – if you have ever experienced back trouble this must be mentioned at your medical. In the exercise section for Back (pages 81-95), high-risk lower back exercises are highlighted and should be avoided if you are a sufferer.

CHASSIS TYPES

Before you begin you ought to coolly assess what is going to be possible for you to achieve. Remember that the key difference between you and a car is that there is no chance of a trade-in for a better or newer model.

Dedication to the exercises set out in this book will achieve results, but they will only improve the body you've got. In order to have a realistic view of what you can achieve it is useful to be aware of the kind of body types available on the open market.

A great deal of confusion arises from the use of some well-known Latin-sounding names for the three classic body-types. These have been disregarded here in favour of more general descriptions of the characteristics you will recognise in the body type most closely resembling yourself.

While your bone structure will always be the same, what hangs on those bones can be subject to dramatic change. Muscles grow through exercise, and reveal or hide themselves through what your body stores as a result of your diet and lifestyle – otherwise known as fat. It is the relationship between muscle and fat and your body's natural ability to control this relationship that has most to do with what you can achieve with the body you've got. A later section deals with eating to reflect your body-improving aims (page 149).

SLIM

Characteristics Bone structure covered by muscle and little else, but natural prominence and definition of muscles is not normal. Natural depth and breadth to the upper body is uncommon.

The good news Fast on your feet, with natural endurance and high energy level. Higher metabolic rate gives you the ability to eat almost anything without ill-effects – provided you *are* exercising. This body type also has the lowest incidence of cardio-vascular disease. Muscular definition is relatively simple.

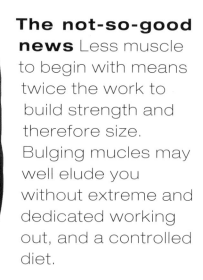

The not-so-good news Less muscle to begin with means twice the work to build strength and therefore size. Bulging mucles may well elude you without extreme and dedicated working out, and a controlled diet.

HUNKY

Characteristics Natural definition to muscles and classically proportioned. Musculature is usually easily visible, with body fat minimal.

The good news Naturally built for sport, muscle responds well to exercise and develops easily. Because body fat is relatively easy to control, definition is most easily achieved for this body type.

The not-so-good news Endurance sports and exercise can be more of an effort as muscle tissue is almost three times the density of fat, which is why swimming is more demanding. Weight gain can sometimes be a problem, especially if you stop exercising after a period of exercise linked to a weight/muscle gain regime.

STOCKY

Characteristics Big and strong, solid in appearance. Muscular definition often softened by higher levels of body fat. Deep upper body and strong lower body are usual.

The good news Muscle can easily be built, which consequently results in above-average strength.

The not-so-good news Larger amounts of body fat mean muscular definition may elude you. Lower metabolic rate means weight gain is a constant concern. Heart disease is also more common, as are weight-bearing joint injuries.

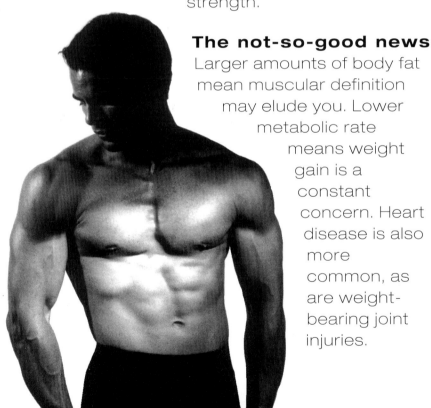

REVS PER MINUTE

All the body-part development exercises in this book are composed of relatively simple movements, which need to be repeated in two different kinds of ways to be effective.

If you have ever been around gym-goers you will have heard the two buzz words <u>reps</u> and <u>sets</u>.

Reps, short (not surprisingly) for repetitions, refers to the number of repeated movements you are able to do at a given weight at any one time. The number of times you can repeat any exercise is of course directly related to the weight you attempt to work with.

Sets refers to the number of times you do a cycle of reps on any one exercise. Although it is largely up to you to determine how many sets you perform, two to three is the norm.

It is the relationship between reps and sets that will largely determine the type of muscular development that will take place in your body.

It is now widely acknowledged that in any one set of reps, working to exhaustion of the muscles involved will result in the most effective workout.

Broadly, **more reps with a lower weight** will result in a more 'endurance working' of the muscles, because you will need to do more reps to get to exhaustion, useful to those seeking to burn fat tissue.

Conversely **fewer reps with a higher weight** will result in a more muscle-building working of the muscles, because what energy you have when working to exhaustion will be concentrated into fewer, more intense reps, useful to those seeking to build muscle mass.

It is for you to determine which route to take, and it may be that you choose different rep/set ratios for different body parts, based on the fact that there may be an imbalance in your body – as there is in most people's – which you may seek to redress by working one body part more aerobically, and another for the building of the relevant muscles

Whichever seems to work for you, you must remember that you are more likely to attain the body you want if your exercise technique is good, as it is all too easy if you are ambitious to **cheat**, or use the **momentum** of an exercise to do more reps than you would be able to do normally. These two are the enemies of results.

Cheating

You will find reference to classic cheats with any of the following exercises where appropriate. Although it may make you feel better to appear to perform the exercise at a higher weight or for more reps, it will be doing no more than if you performed it properly.

Momentum

This is where the natural 'swing' of any exercise is utilized to complete a rep. The exercise illustrated below is a classic example of when it is possible to complete a higher number of reps by swinging the dumbells up to the shoulder. In this exercise the only body parts which should move are the lower arms. Concentrate on the body part being exercised, and make sure that it is the only place you can feel exertion.

This will be the simplest way to guarantee the quality and effectiveness of your workout programme.

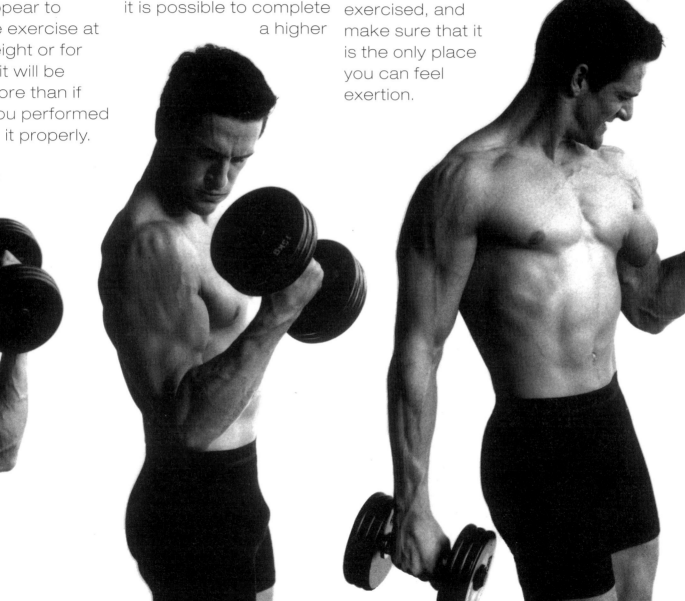

WORKSHOP ROUTINE

Of course no results will be achieved without actually visiting the gym and working out, and allocating time in your life to do this may be the most difficult part of embarking on your body-improving programme. Not breaking the discipline of going to the gym is a key part of the dedication you will have to display if your routine is to be effective.

There is no evidence to prove that there is any particular benefit in working out at any specific time of day, so choose your preferred time **and stick to it**.

The exercises in this book are contained in five coloured sections:

Green	Warm-up & stretch	pages 23-31
Yellow	Chest	pages 33-47
	Shoulders	pages 49-63
Orange	Legs	pages 65-79
	Back	pages 81-95
Red	Arms	pages 97-111
	Abdominals	pages 113-127
Blue	Cool-down	pages 129-137

A personal programme should be constructed as follows:

DAY ONE	DAY TWO
Green	
Cardio of your choice	Different cardio
Stretch selection	Different stretch
Yellow	
Chest selection	Shoulder selection
Orange	
Leg selection	Back selection
Red	
Arm selection	Abdominal selection
Blue	
Reverse cardio	Different rev. cardio
Cool-down selection	Different cool-down

This two-day split could be applied to two trips per week, or four per week. Alternatively, working out every other day – or every day – is simply a question of keeping a track of which day routine you did last. A six-day cycle with one body part from yellow, orange and red is another variation.

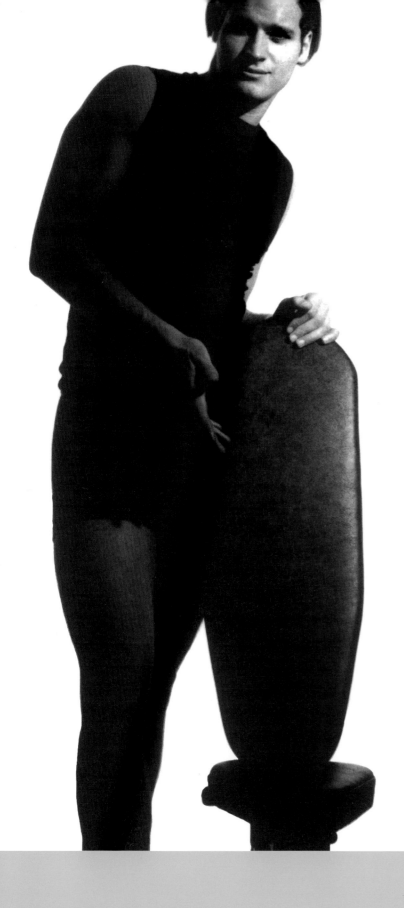

GOLDEN RULES

Never work the same body part twice in 24 hours – in other words, don't do chest two days running, for example.

Try to vary the exercises you do for each body part between the last time you did it and the next. The body can get attuned to what is expected of it and this may be one of the key points at which momentum and cheating can most easily sneak into your routine.

Don't skip your cardio warm-up or stretch – starting a car from cold and going from 0-60 isn't a good idea and this applies to the human body too.

Give yourself at least one day off a week and don't get into the state of mind that leaving off your workout – say for a holiday – will result in deterioration. Your body will definitely benefit from rest and relaxation, and coming back refreshed to an exercise regimen is always good.

No matter how confident you feel about going to the gym for the first time after reading this book, do make use of the induction programme (free in all gyms) that you will be offered, and ask for additional exercises for body parts you particularly want to improve – good instructors know them all.

Don't ignore the advice of gym instructors – they've seen every kind of technique and mistake so anything they say about how to do exercises should be listened to.

COMMON DAMAGE

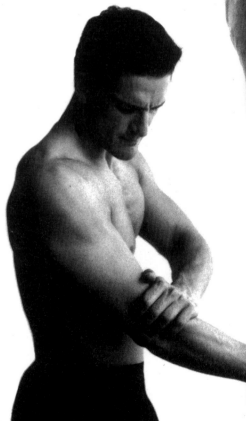

To understand something about what your body will be going through when you embark on a weight-training programme, the slightly gruesome truth about muscle growth must now be revealed.

When you lift weights during exercise and work the muscle concerned to exhaustion, the burn that you will feel if you are doing it right is the pain caused by muscle tissue damage and the body's natural defences rushing to aid repair.

Miraculously it is able to perform these repairs in record time – hence the need to leave 24 hours between working the same body part again.

It is the constant cycle of muscle tissue damage and repair that builds muscle mass, since the body is actually adjusting the size and strength of muscles in line with the new levels of strain being placed on them on a regular basis.

Not only is there the pain of the original burn to deal with, but during the repair period itself you should feel aching if the exercises you have performed have been effective at all.

Initially, especially if you throw yourself wholeheartedly into your gym programme, you will feel practically crippled with an overall muscular ache. As your body rapidly adjusts to compensate, this will ease on a daily basis, but you will notice revisited intensity of pain after a period away from training.

As a general rule, muscular pain brought on from exercise is normal and to be tolerated, and since you work evenly on both sides of the body the ache you notice should also be even across the body.

The isolation of an ache or a sharper pain may be an indication of something more serious, such as a strained tendon, or maladjustment of muscle groups through overworking your favourite muscle group. **Seek medical advice if you notice pain of this kind.** A trip to the gym osteopath may be an expense worth affording.

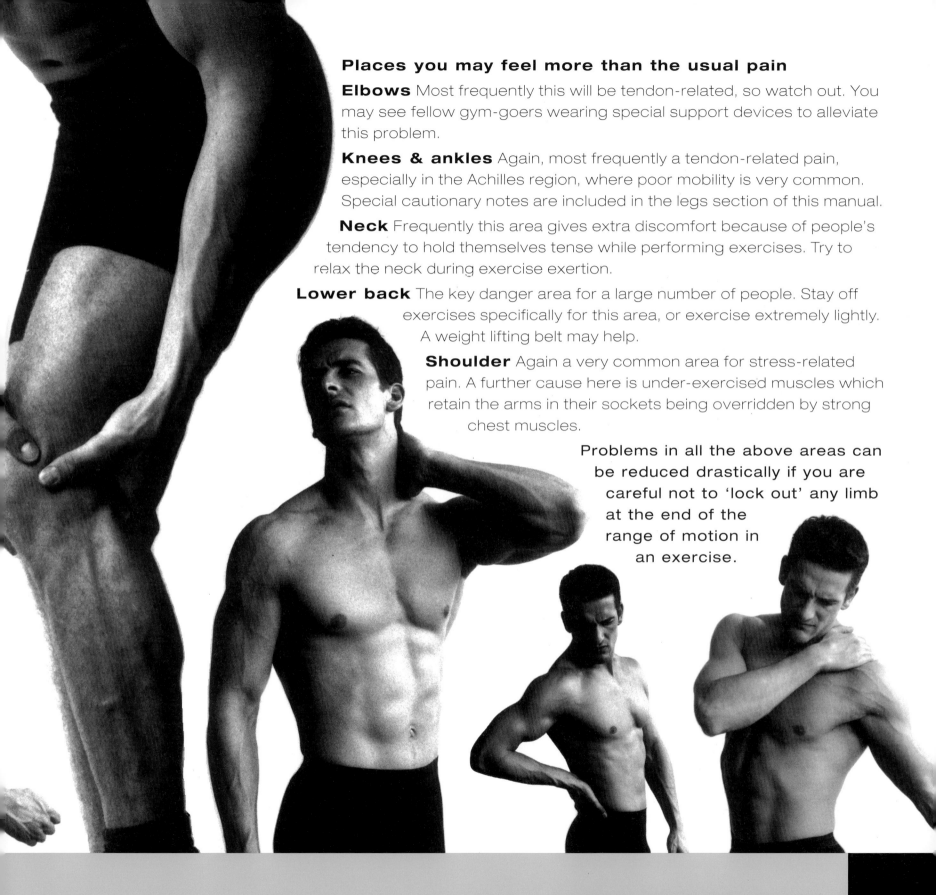

Places you may feel more than the usual pain

Elbows Most frequently this will be tendon-related, so watch out. You may see fellow gym-goers wearing special support devices to alleviate this problem.

Knees & ankles Again, most frequently a tendon-related pain, especially in the Achilles region, where poor mobility is very common. Special cautionary notes are included in the legs section of this manual.

Neck Frequently this area gives extra discomfort because of people's tendency to hold themselves tense while performing exercises. Try to relax the neck during exercise exertion.

Lower back The key danger area for a large number of people. Stay off exercises specifically for this area, or exercise extremely lightly. A weight lifting belt may help.

Shoulder Again a very common area for stress-related pain. A further cause here is under-exercised muscles which retain the arms in their sockets being overridden by strong chest muscles.

Problems in all the above areas can be reduced drastically if you are careful not to 'lock out' any limb at the end of the range of motion in an exercise.

MINOR REPAIRS

Unfortunately, any aching pain you feel when you begin a gym programme will have to be put up with, but you may find it helpful at first to leave longer between workouts to let the ache subside.

The term 'muscle-bound' can come to apply if proper care is not taken to ensure full mobility around your joints. Aerobic exercise during warm-up and stretch exercises can help, but professional sportsmen also draw on other methods to aid healthy muscle condition, and joint and tendon mobility.

Such methods can also mean that you do not have to suffer in silence with the general aches and pains of muscle development. The treatments involved are not unpleasureable.

Sauna Many gyms have a sauna in the changing area, and the action of dry heat on a wet body – optionally enhanced by the passage-clearing properties of pine-impregnated water applied to the open heat source – can be particularly effective in the relaxation of muscles tensed by an intensive workout.

If you can stand it, the original Finnish method involves taking an ice-cold shower between visits to the sauna cubicle. This is reputed to be to energize the body and skin, but in practice it is to enable you to tolerate the heat of the sauna for a longer period without ill-effect.

Steam room Less common, but often an alternative to the sauna, the steam room is literally that – a room filled with steam.

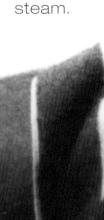

The same therapeutic benefits are ascribed to the steam room as the sauna, and its key benefit is that people who find the sauna too extreme are able to tolerate the generally (slightly) cooler atmosphere.

Cold showers or a plunge-pool as part of the treatment are the authentic Turkish method.

Massage All gyms can now arrange to put you in touch with masseurs of all kinds, but the most effective for weight-training gym-goers is deep tissue massage of the type used by sportsmen.

Most gyms now also have the benefit of their own treatment rooms, which can mean that a relaxing and beneficial massage can follow immediately after a workout. Massage treatment is not cheap, but it should be borne in mind what very hard physical work it is for your masseur. It is good value.

The osteopath For a persistent or isolated ache or pain, this may be the answer. Trained in the art of muscle and joint manipulation, the freeing of poorly-mobilised areas of the body is the osteopath's speciality.

Again, it may be possible to see an osteopath in the treatment room of your gym.

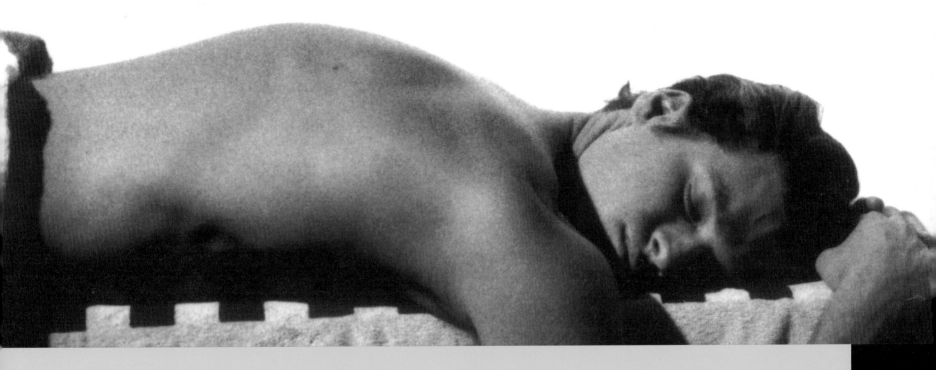

OVERALLS

What you wear in the gym is entirely up to you, but there are a few aspects of this subject which must be discussed as they have implications for safety or comfort.

The models performing the exercises in this book are dressed so that you can see the movements they are performing most clearly, but certain gyms have strict dress codes which would, for example, make the wearing of a top compulsory.

The subject of personal hygiene needs to also be raised at this point: you will not be the most popular member of the gym if you work out in the same outfit all week.

You should also consider the risk of foot disease, and many people now wear flip-flops in the shower area to avoid the transmission of such conditions.

Shoes It is obvious when you visit a sports shoe store that the choice now offered is very wide, but many are less suitable for the gym. Look for the following in your selection:

Suppleness *Calf exercises require flexibility for full foot movement*

Protection *Remember that you might drop weights*

Support *The ankle and the Achilles tendon are weak*

Gloves You may find the knurled grips of free weights produce hard-skin areas which weight-training gloves help to alleviate. Gloves extending over the wrist also afford some support.

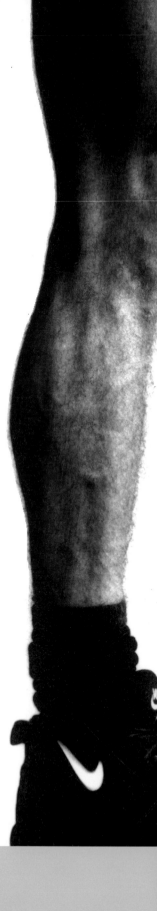

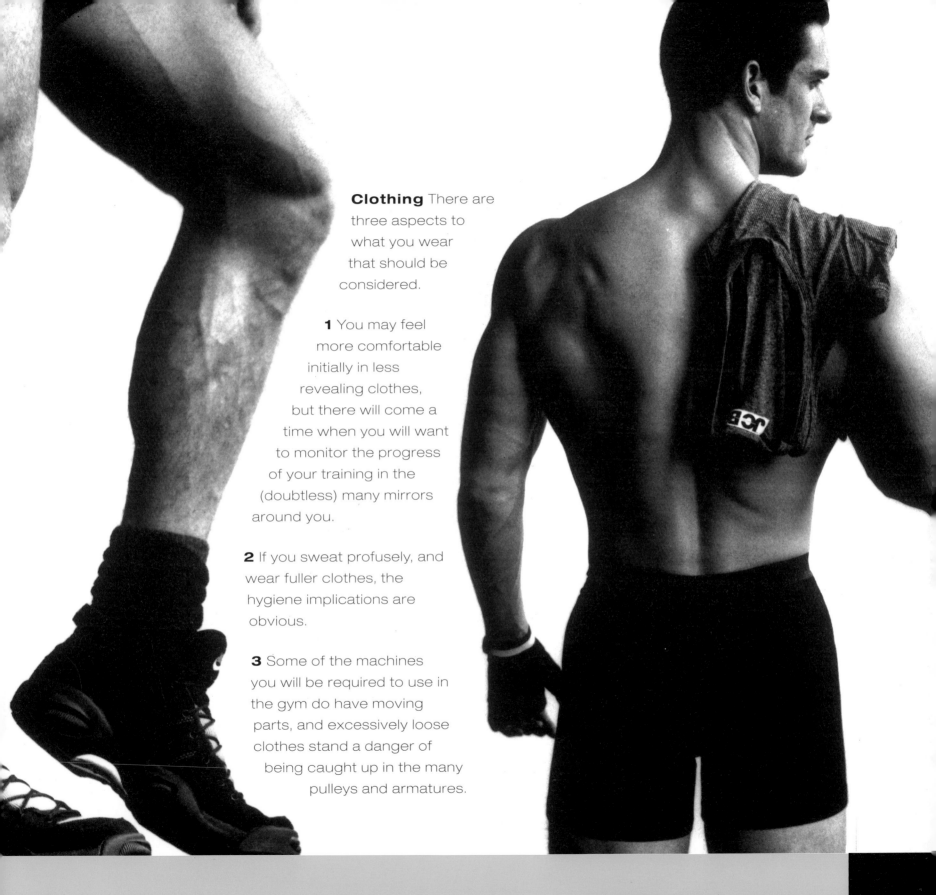

Clothing There are three aspects to what you wear that should be considered.

1 You may feel more comfortable initially in less revealing clothes, but there will come a time when you will want to monitor the progress of your training in the (doubtless) many mirrors around you.

2 If you sweat profusely, and wear fuller clothes, the hygiene implications are obvious.

3 Some of the machines you will be required to use in the gym do have moving parts, and excessively loose clothes stand a danger of being caught up in the many pulleys and armatures.

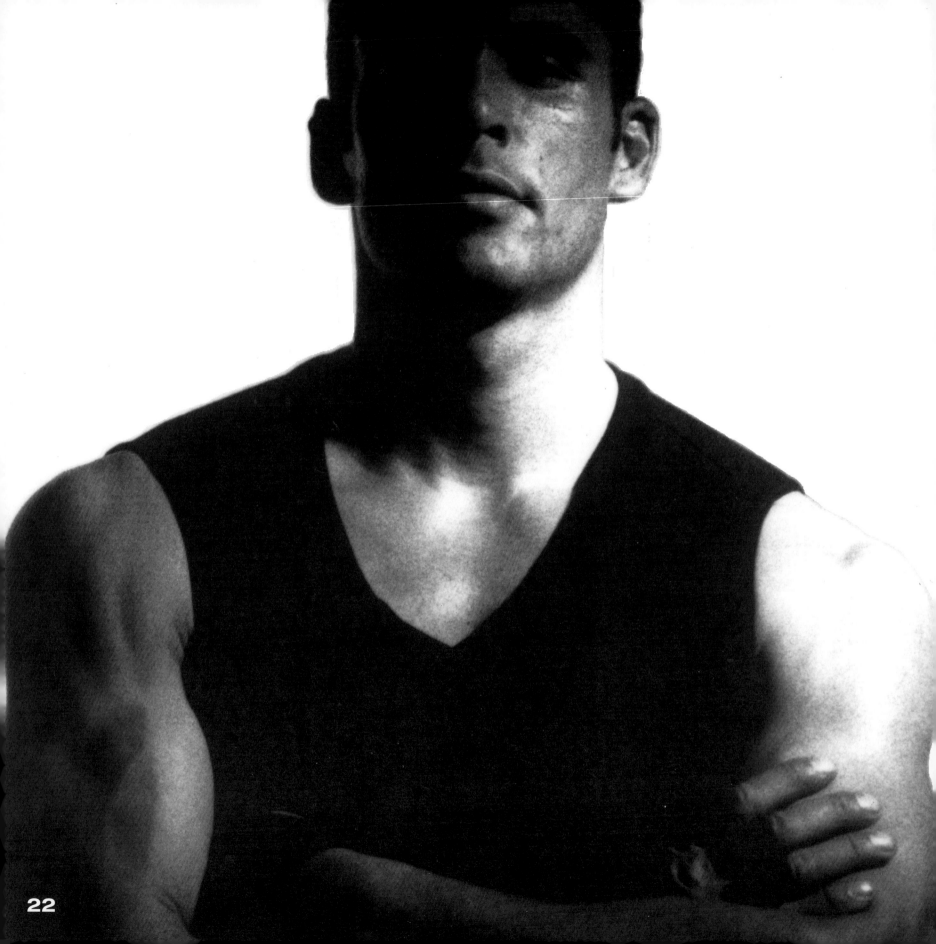

So you're in the door and ready to start – now what? Before you begin the specific muscle group exercises, it's time to build up a bit of a sweat and get those joints moving freely.

IGNITION

Exercises from the following section should be performed on every occasion you visit the gym – or you may live to regret it!

Section essentials

Never start a workout session from cold.

Always start with cardio-vascular exercise.

Do not rest too long after cardio-vascular exercise – your body should not be allowed to cool down.

Do not hold the stretch exercise positions (pages 26-31) for longer than the count of eight as this will also encourage your body to cool down.

If you choose to skip cardio-vascular work at the gym because you have cycled or run to the gym do not skip your stretch exercises.

Breathe freely and deeply during cardio-vascular exercise.

Do not hold your breath during a stretch exercise – breathe normally.

ACCELERATION

When you are in a hurry it is all too tempting to skip this important warm-up process, and get straight into the muscle-building exercises. But don't – it has been remarked before that cars don't perform best straight from cold, and the body doesn't either.

All gyms have a good range of cardio-vascular (heart/blood-energizing) machines, which are convenient, stationary versions of pursuits you would otherwise perform outside.

If you live or work near your gym you could replace this warm-up by actually jogging or cycling there.

Otherwise, ten minutes on any of the cardio machines will suffice to build up your body temperature and heart rate. Longer than this will be useful to those with a need to reduce body fat, as aerobic exercise of this sort is a natural energy burner.

Rowing machine

Simulates the workout you would get on your local river in a skiff, but without the risk of capsizing. A good workout for the shoulders prior to working that body part, it is also one of the better all-round warm-up machines. Different resistance levels can be adjusted to increase your workload, but the work intensity is determined by your stroke speed.

Running machine

Otherwise known as the treadmill, some complain that it is a poor substitute for the real thing, but as you are not at risk of foul weather or collision with other people or vehicles it does have its plus points. The fancier models can incline so that you are running uphill, and speeds can be pre-set for a thorough warm-up or aerobic workout.

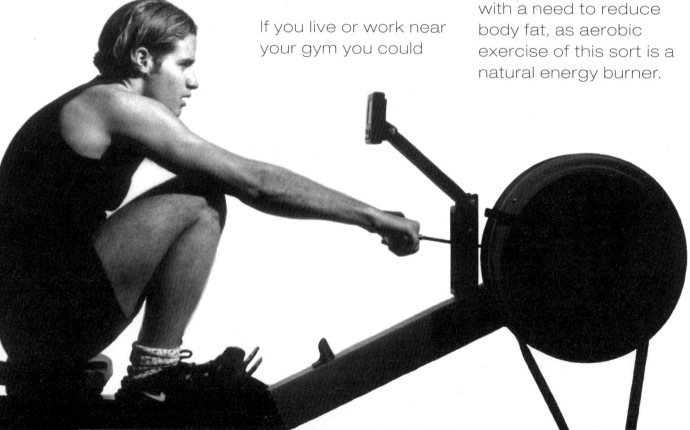

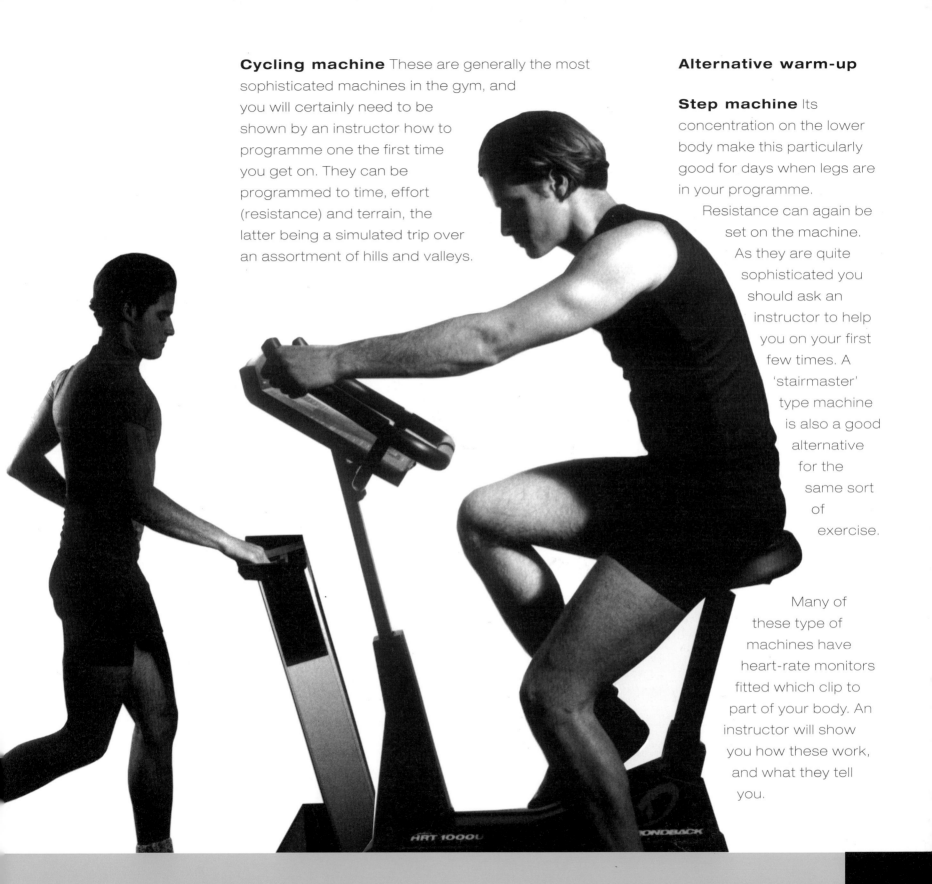

Cycling machine These are generally the most sophisticated machines in the gym, and you will certainly need to be shown by an instructor how to programme one the first time you get on. They can be programmed to time, effort (resistance) and terrain, the latter being a simulated trip over an assortment of hills and valleys.

Alternative warm-up

Step machine Its concentration on the lower body make this particularly good for days when legs are in your programme.

Resistance can again be set on the machine. As they are quite sophisticated you should ask an instructor to help you on your first few times. A 'stairmaster' type machine is also a good alternative for the same sort of exercise.

Many of these type of machines have heart-rate monitors fitted which clip to part of your body. An instructor will show you how these work, and what they tell you.

HRT 1000U

CHANGING GEAR

Although there is no conclusive evidence to support the theory that stretching before exercise can help prevent injury, it is still a good idea to pick a selection of the exercises in this section to perform before you start your workout.

Side bends With legs on a wide base, knees bent, and the left hand behind the head **1**, and with the right on your right thigh supporting the upper body on the right side, bend to your right straight down the bodyline as far as you can, ensuring you do not twist **2**. Hold for the count of eight, then relax. Feel the stretch from armpit to waist. Repeat, but this time with the right hand behind the head **3**, bending to your left. Use either of the two supporting hand positions shown – whichever is most comfortable for you.

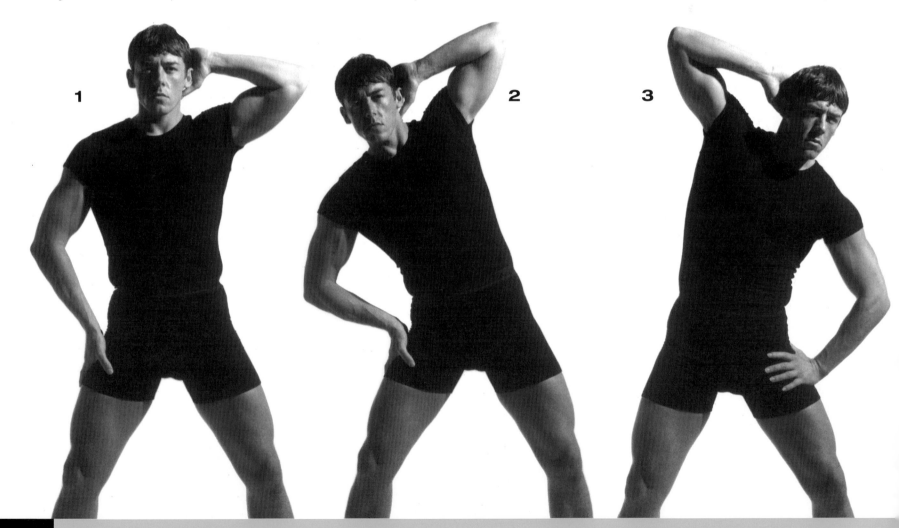

Torso stretch Standing, with straight back, raise your arms to the sky and then raise yourself on tiptoe. Feel the stretch from your shoulders down to your waist. Hold for the count of eight, then relax.

Foot-forward hamstring stretch Standing, with your left foot forward but not locked straight, and with your heel on the floor and your foot at right-angles, lean forward **1**, keeping your back straight, **2**. Your right foot should be flat on the ground, with your right knee bent, and it is essential that your upper body is supported by your hands on your right thigh to protect the lower back from injury. Feel the stretch right down the back of your left leg. Hold for the count of twenty, then relax. Repeat with the right leg.

The hamstring is the muscle running down the back of your leg.

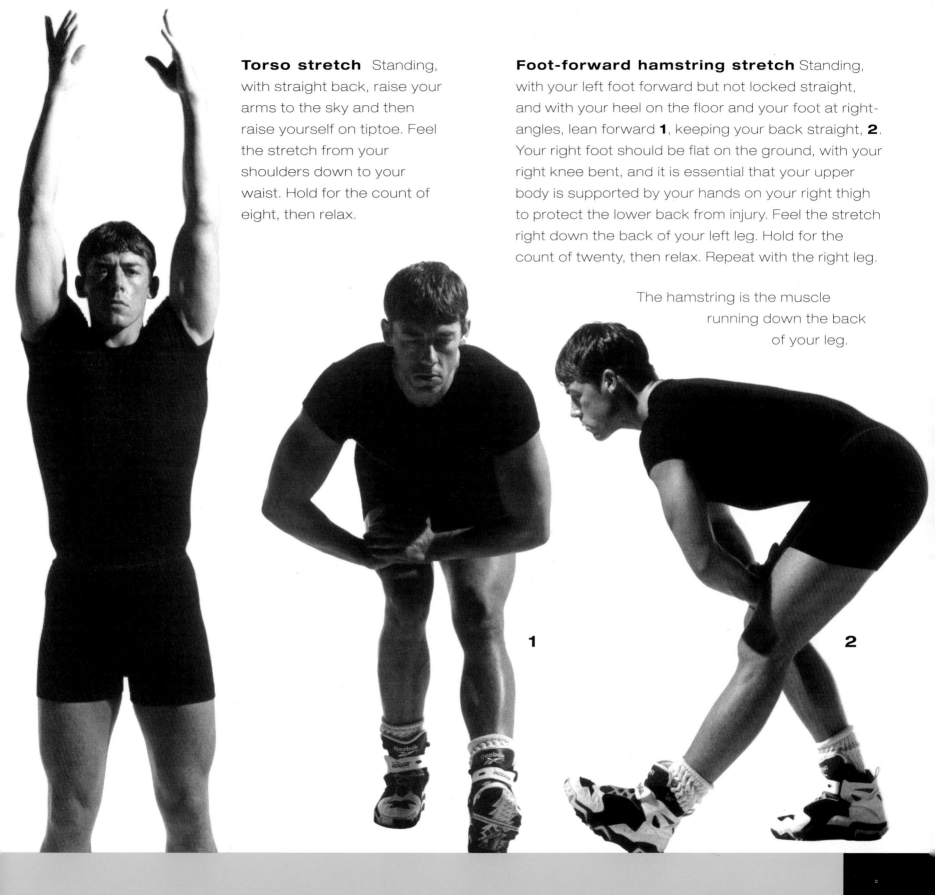

1

2

Shoulder stretch Standing, with straight back, knees slightly bent, stomach pulled in, reach across your body with your right arm. Bring your left hand to just above your right elbow and gently press the arm across your body, **1**. Feel the stretch strongly concentrate in your shoulder. Hold for the count of eight, then relax.

Repeat with the left arm **2**, pressing above the left elbow with the right hand across the body.

This should not give you discomfort in your elbow – check your technique if this is the case.

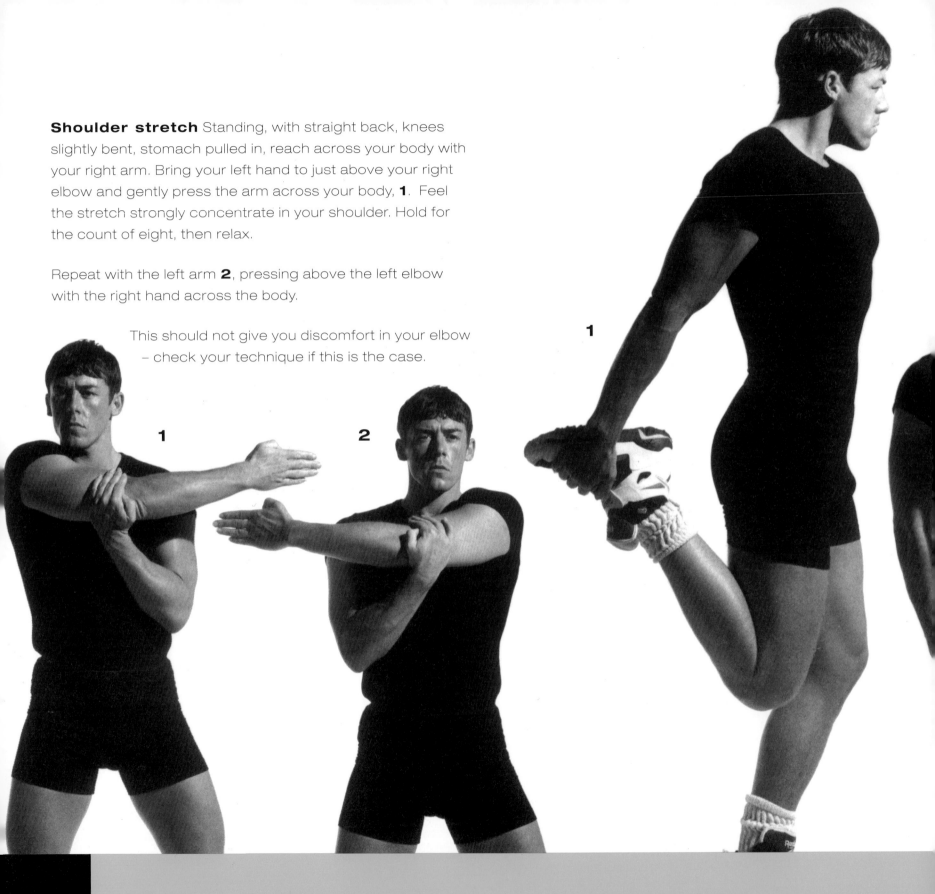

Standing quad stretch Standing, with straight back, knees slightly bent and stomach pulled in, raise your right foot to meet your right hand. Holding your right foot, gently pull towards the right buttock – but stop a few inches short of touching **1**. Hold the leg back, and press the right hip forward, by tilting your pelvis under. Feel the stretch down the front of your thigh. Hold for the count of twenty, then relax.

Repeat with the left leg, held with the left hand **2**.

The quads are the large muscles you can feel if you tense your thigh when it is raised to the horizontal when you are seated.

Pectoral stretch With both hands linked behind your back, fingers intertwined or resting on top of each other, palms upward **1**, draw shoulders back, attempting to bring elbows together **2**. Feel the stretch from your shoulder across the top of your chest, **3**. Take care not to arch your lower back. Hold for the count of eight, then relax.

The pectorals are the large plate-like muscles on the front of your chest.

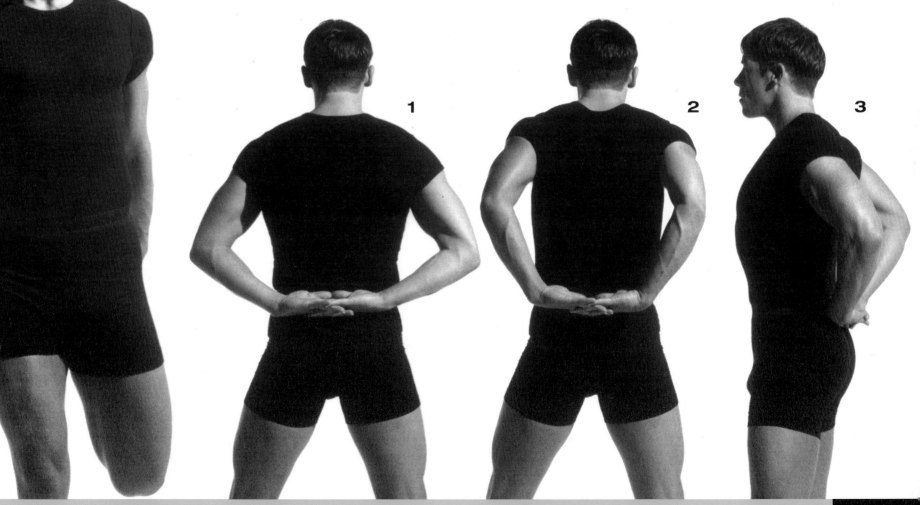

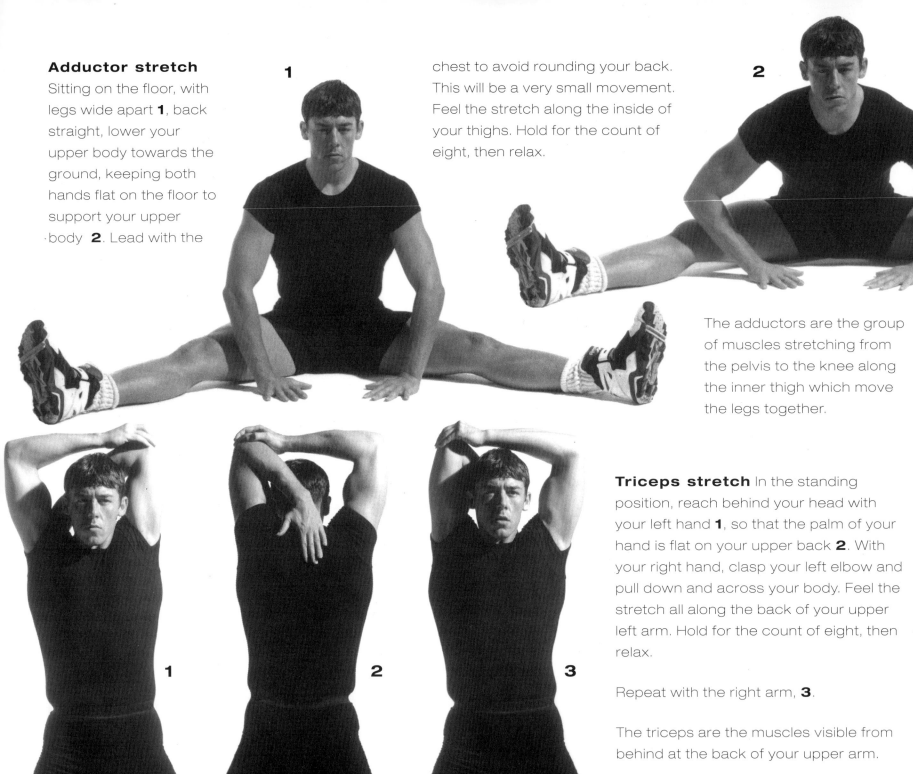

Adductor stretch

Sitting on the floor, with legs wide apart **1**, back straight, lower your upper body towards the ground, keeping both hands flat on the floor to support your upper body **2**. Lead with the chest to avoid rounding your back. This will be a very small movement. Feel the stretch along the inside of your thighs. Hold for the count of eight, then relax.

The adductors are the group of muscles stretching from the pelvis to the knee along the inner thigh which move the legs together.

Triceps stretch

In the standing position, reach behind your head with your left hand **1**, so that the palm of your hand is flat on your upper back **2**. With your right hand, clasp your left elbow and pull down and across your body. Feel the stretch all along the back of your upper left arm. Hold for the count of eight, then relax.

Repeat with the right arm, **3**.

The triceps are the muscles visible from behind at the back of your upper arm.

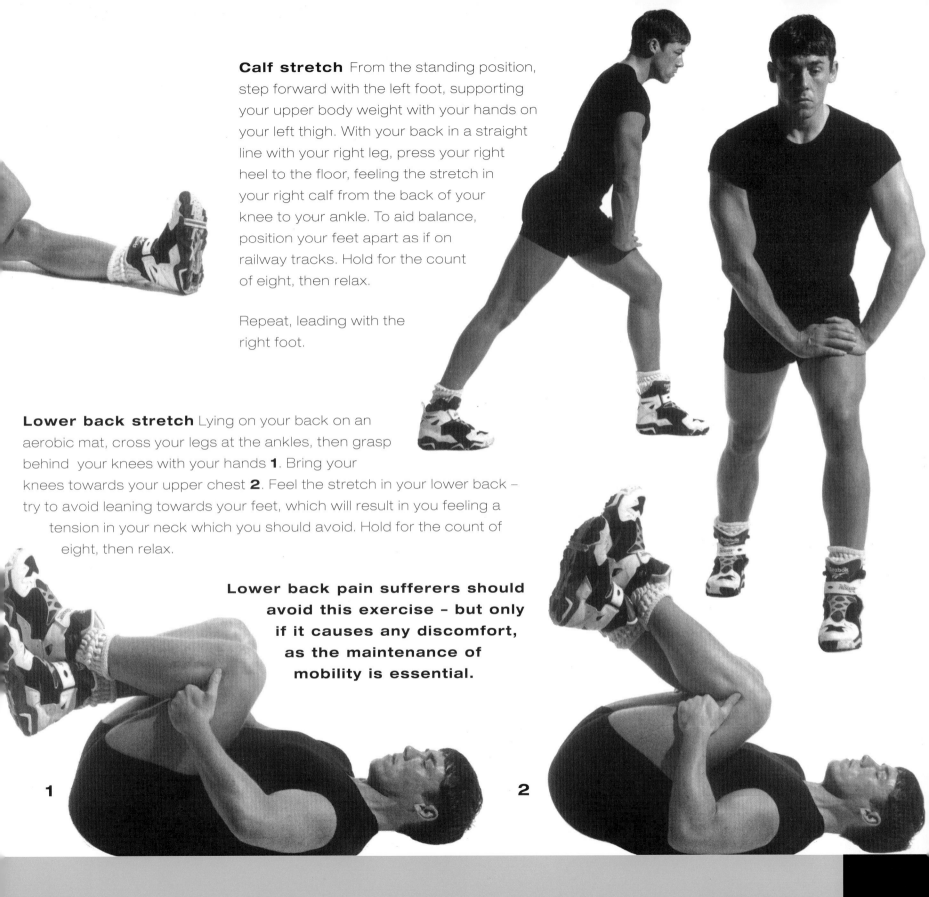

Calf stretch From the standing position, step forward with the left foot, supporting your upper body weight with your hands on your left thigh. With your back in a straight line with your right leg, press your right heel to the floor, feeling the stretch in your right calf from the back of your knee to your ankle. To aid balance, position your feet apart as if on railway tracks. Hold for the count of eight, then relax.

Repeat, leading with the right foot.

Lower back stretch Lying on your back on an aerobic mat, cross your legs at the ankles, then grasp behind your knees with your hands **1**. Bring your knees towards your upper chest **2**. Feel the stretch in your lower back – try to avoid leaning towards your feet, which will result in you feeling a tension in your neck which you should avoid. Hold for the count of eight, then relax.

Lower back pain sufferers should avoid this exercise – but only if it causes any discomfort, as the maintenance of mobility is essential.

1

2

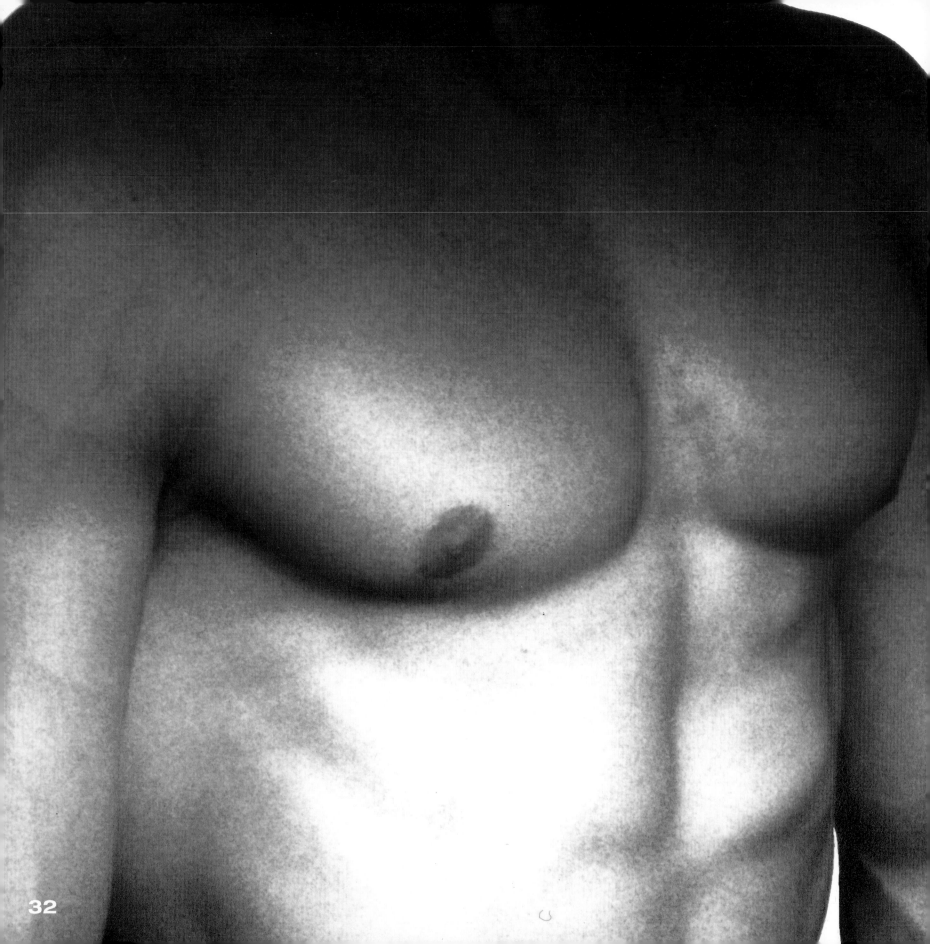

Giving shape and depth to the upper body, the chest area – and its definition – has come to assume an importance for some gym-goers that almost ranks with the significance of the same area in women.

SERVICING OF MOVING PARTS **CHEST**

The large plate-like muscles that sit on the top of the rib cage are the **pectorals**. These are the main focus for the exercises for this body area.

Section essentials

All exercises should be performed to exhaustion, i.e. to the point at which you cannot achieve another rep.

The weight selected should be chosen to achieve the following ratio of reps and sets for *either*

Endurance work:
2–3 sets of 15–20 reps

or

Muscle building work:
3–5 sets of 6–8 reps

Rest between sets for only the length of time it has taken you to perform the previous set.

Take a deep breath prior to starting an exercise, then exhale on the exertion and inhale on the recovery. Do not hold your breath – this may dangerously elevate the blood pressure.

Where your arms or legs are working towards being straight, take care not to 'lock out'. Keep limbs slightly bent.

Explore possibilities beyond the exercises shown. Ask for instruction on isolation machines available for specific body parts that you can add into your programme for variety.

The key basic exercises for the chest are done on **press benches**, for which there are a few important, not-to-be-overlooked, guidelines.

When exhaustion is reached in chest presses, you will be on an upward movement, at the full extent of which you will be replacing the bar on the hooks of the machine. If you do reach exhaustion only part way to the top of this upward movement, the tendency will be to let the bar drop down again.

Obviously, the upper chest and neck are particularly vulnerable from injury should you drop the bar.

For this reason, many people choose to perform all three bench presses with a 'spotter' – a friend or an instructor briefed to catch the bar and assist you to reach exhaustion, and to help replace the bar. Alternatively, you can use a <u>Smith machine</u> if you are on your own, because you can hook the bar back onto the machine at any point. This is probably safest option for beginner's bench pressing.

For some reason the press benches are the most annoying of any of the gym machines to arrive at and find still loaded from the previous user. If you want to make friends at your gym, re-stack your <u>plates</u>.

Basic bench press Before you perform this exercise for the first time, practise the movement with an unloaded bar, and only load the bar with suitable plates when you are confident with the movement, and your hand and body positions. Always err on the side of caution, and start light.

Lie on your back, with your head comfortably supported at the end of the bench, and your feet firmly on the floor, shoulder distance apart. Your eyes should be directly under the bar as it sits on the rack.

2

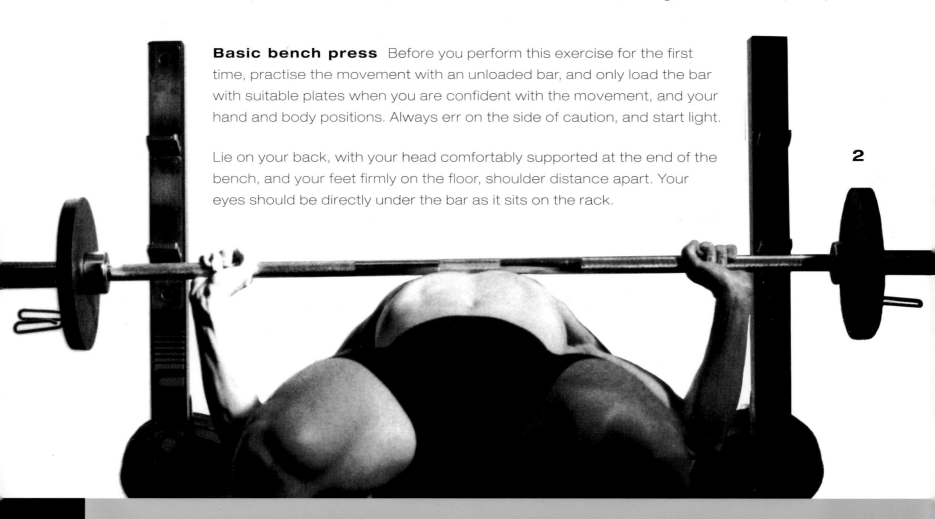

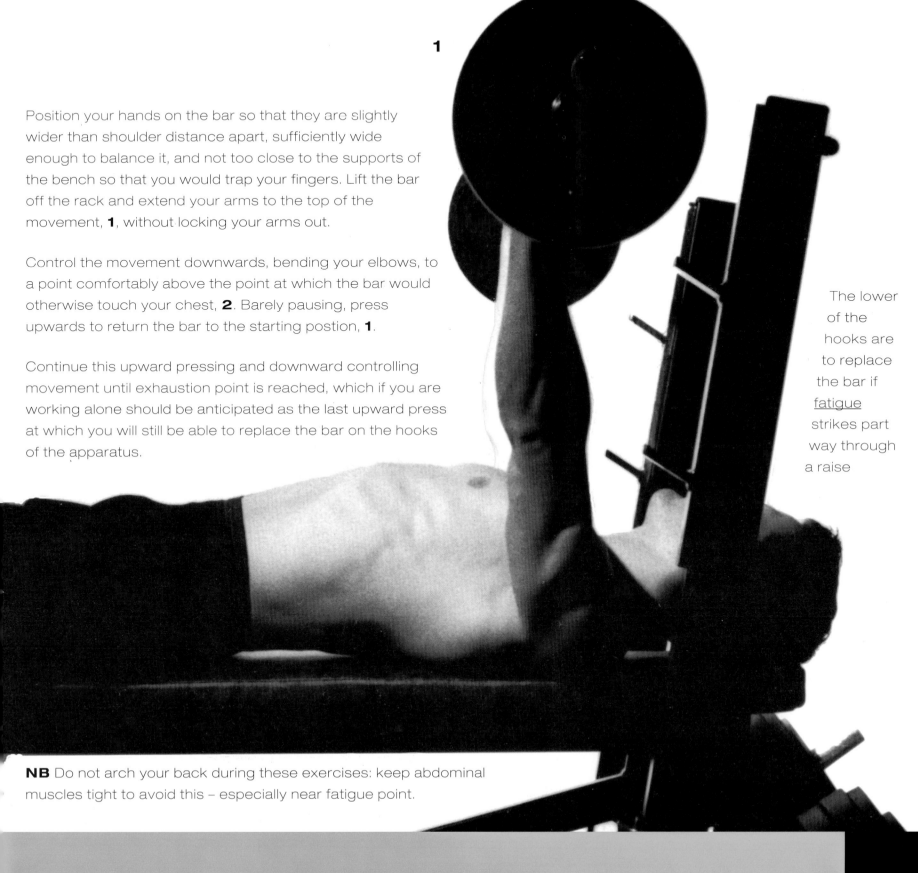

Position your hands on the bar so that they are slightly wider than shoulder distance apart, sufficiently wide enough to balance it, and not too close to the supports of the bench so that you would trap your fingers. Lift the bar off the rack and extend your arms to the top of the movement, **1**, without locking your arms out.

Control the movement downwards, bending your elbows, to a point comfortably above the point at which the bar would otherwise touch your chest, **2**. Barely pausing, press upwards to return the bar to the starting postion, **1**.

Continue this upward pressing and downward controlling movement until exhaustion point is reached, which if you are working alone should be anticipated as the last upward press at which you will still be able to replace the bar on the hooks of the apparatus.

The lower of the hooks are to replace the bar if <u>fatigue</u> strikes part way through a raise

NB Do not arch your back during these exercises: keep abdominal muscles tight to avoid this – especially near fatigue point.

Incline bench press Again, before you perform this exercise for the first time, practise the movement with an unloaded bar. The action is subtly different from the basic bench press.

Lie back on the bench, with your head and body supported, and your feet firmly on the floor, shoulder distance apart. Your forehead should be directly under the bar when it is on its hooks.

Position your hands on the bar wider apart than for the basic bench press, but still far enough away from the supports to avoid trapping your hands. Lift the bar off and extend your arms to the top of the movement, **1**, without locking your arms out.

Control the movement down to a point slightly above actual contact with your chest, **2**. Without pausing, return the bar to the top of the movement, without jerking and with a consistent, smooth action.

Repeat to exhaustion, replacing the bar at the top of your last repetition.

If you do enlist the services of a 'spotter' there is usually a platform on which they can stand, from where they can assist you.

1

2

NB Do not arch your back during these exercises: keep abdominal muscles tight to avoid this – especially near fatigue point.

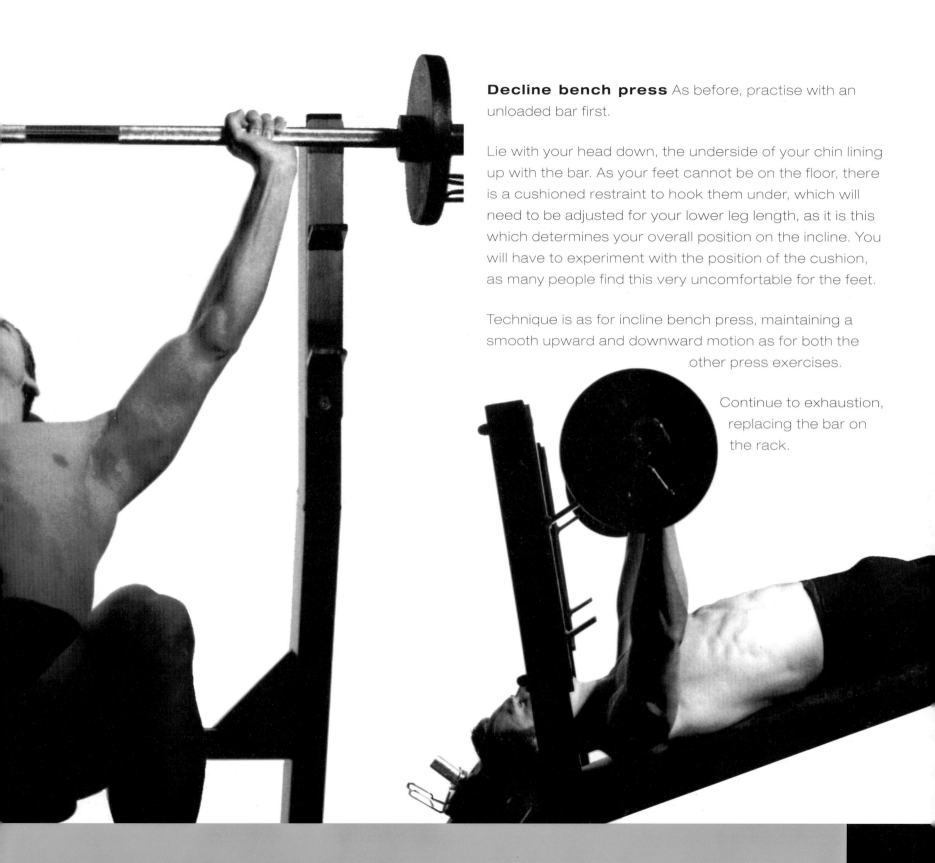

Decline bench press As before, practise with an unloaded bar first.

Lie with your head down, the underside of your chin lining up with the bar. As your feet cannot be on the floor, there is a cushioned restraint to hook them under, which will need to be adjusted for your lower leg length, as it is this which determines your overall position on the incline. You will have to experiment with the position of the cushion, as many people find this very uncomfortable for the feet.

Technique is as for incline bench press, maintaining a smooth upward and downward motion as for both the other press exercises.

Continue to exhaustion, replacing the bar on the rack.

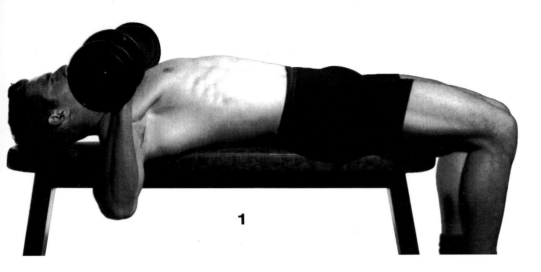

1

Flat dumb-bell press Essentially the same movement as the basic bench press, but without the restriction of the hands staying a fixed distance apart, which means the inner parts of the pectorals are worked.

Select a pair of suitable dumb-bells, then sit and lie back on a flat bench. Use the momentum of lying back to swing the dumb-bells to the starting position, **1**, postioned above where arm meets shoulder, feet firmly on the floor.

Press upwards, bringing dumb-bells to meet, flat side to flat side, above your chest, **2**, without locking out. Control the movement down smoothly.

Continue the movement to exhaustion. There is a knack to getting up from this exercise. Resting the dumb-bells on your chest, raise your knees towards your chest, and then swing down again to the floor with your legs, using the momentum to aid you in sitting up, bringing the dumb-bells to rest on your thighs.

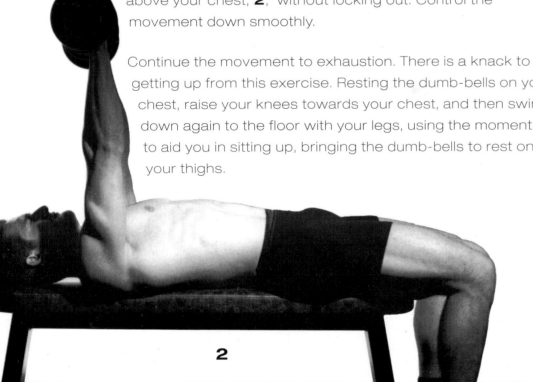

2

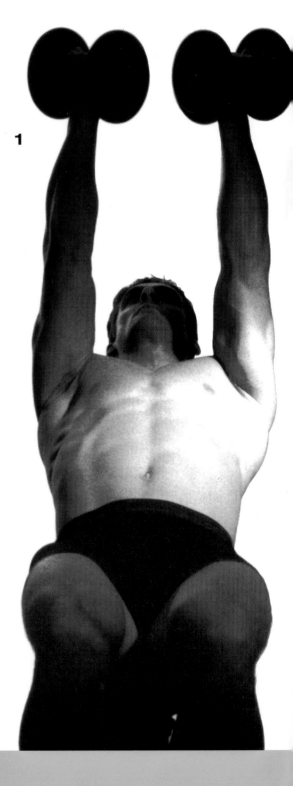

1

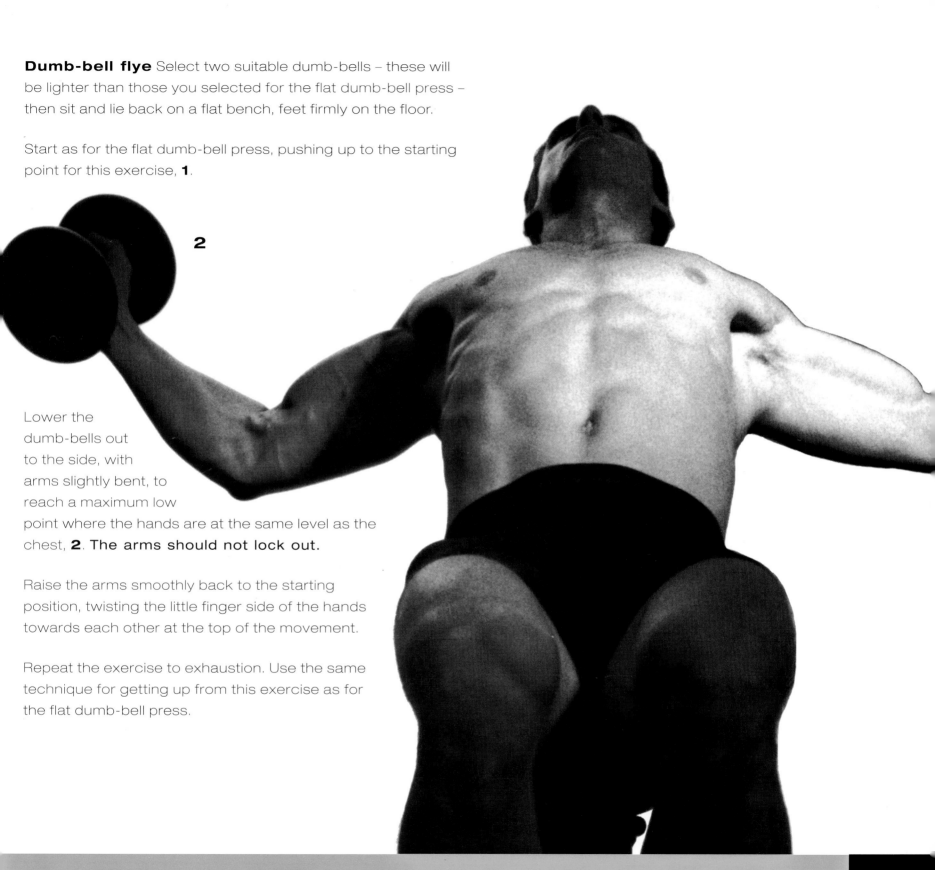

Dumb-bell flye Select two suitable dumb-bells – these will be lighter than those you selected for the flat dumb-bell press – then sit and lie back on a flat bench, feet firmly on the floor.

Start as for the flat dumb-bell press, pushing up to the starting point for this exercise, **1**.

2

Lower the dumb-bells out to the side, with arms slightly bent, to reach a maximum low point where the hands are at the same level as the chest, **2**. The arms should not lock out.

Raise the arms smoothly back to the starting position, twisting the little finger side of the hands towards each other at the top of the movement.

Repeat the exercise to exhaustion. Use the same technique for getting up from this exercise as for the flat dumb-bell press.

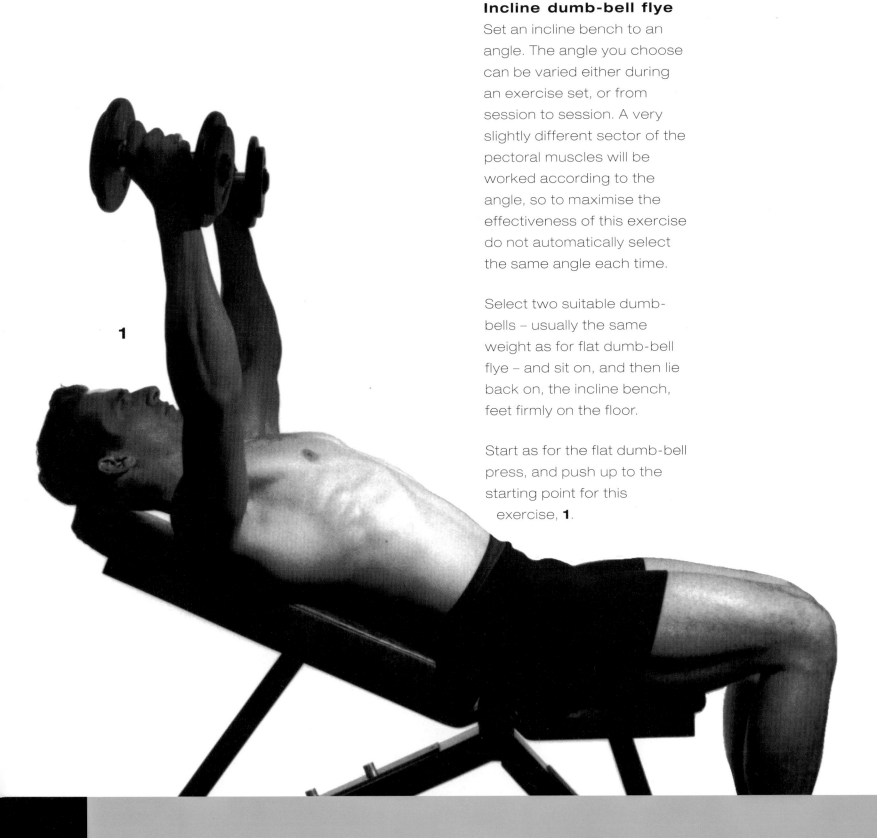

Incline dumb-bell flye

Set an incline bench to an angle. The angle you choose can be varied either during an exercise set, or from session to session. A very slightly different sector of the pectoral muscles will be worked according to the angle, so to maximise the effectiveness of this exercise do not automatically select the same angle each time.

Select two suitable dumb-bells – usually the same weight as for flat dumb-bell flye – and sit on, and then lie back on, the incline bench, feet firmly on the floor.

Start as for the flat dumb-bell press, and push up to the starting point for this exercise, **1**.

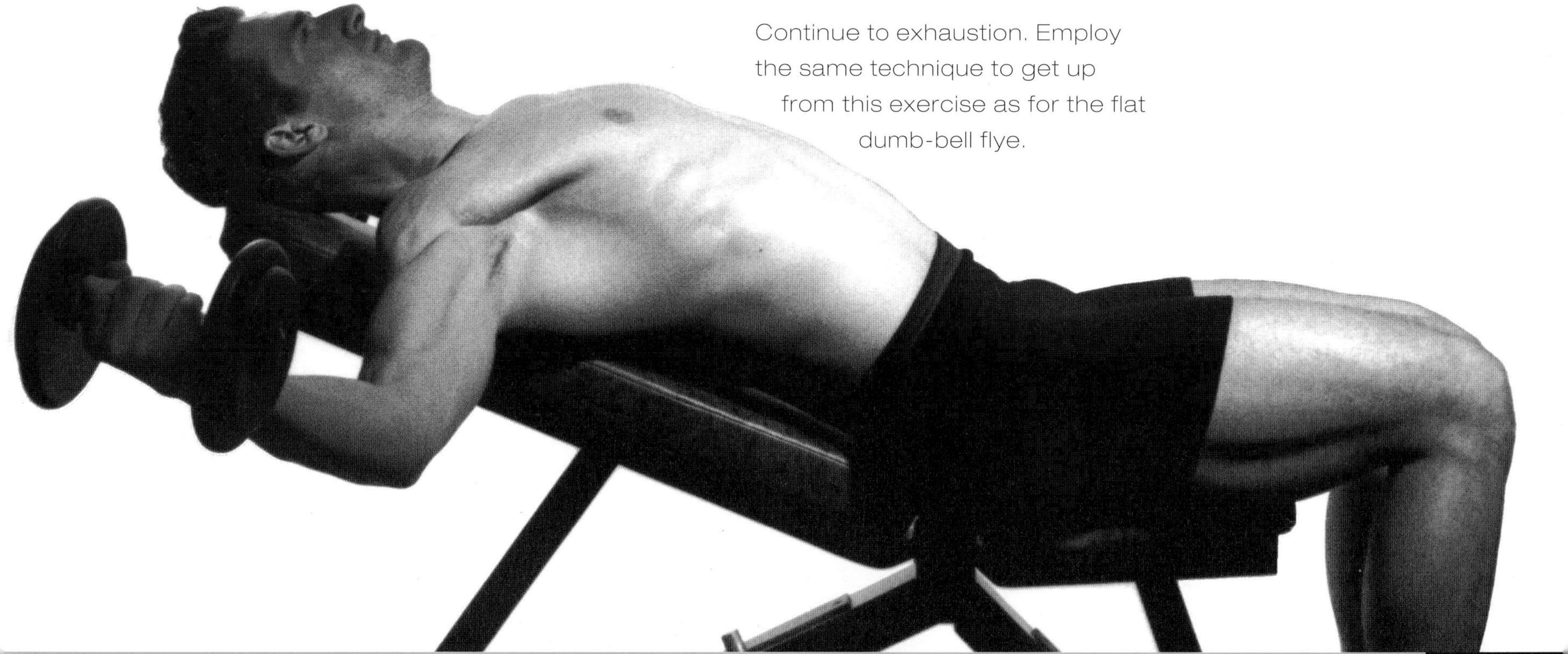

Lower the dumb-bells out to the side, with arms slightly bent, working to the full range of comfortable movement for you, **2**. **The arms should not lock out.**

Raise the weights smoothly back to the top of the movement, rotating the wrists slightly to bring the little finger side of the hands together. The rotation increases the effectiveness of this exercise, and you will feel this in the centre of the chest as the pectorals flex towards each other.

Arms should be slightly bent throughout the exercise.

Continue to exhaustion. Employ the same technique to get up from this exercise as for the flat dumb-bell flye.

2

INCLINE DUMB-BELL FLYE

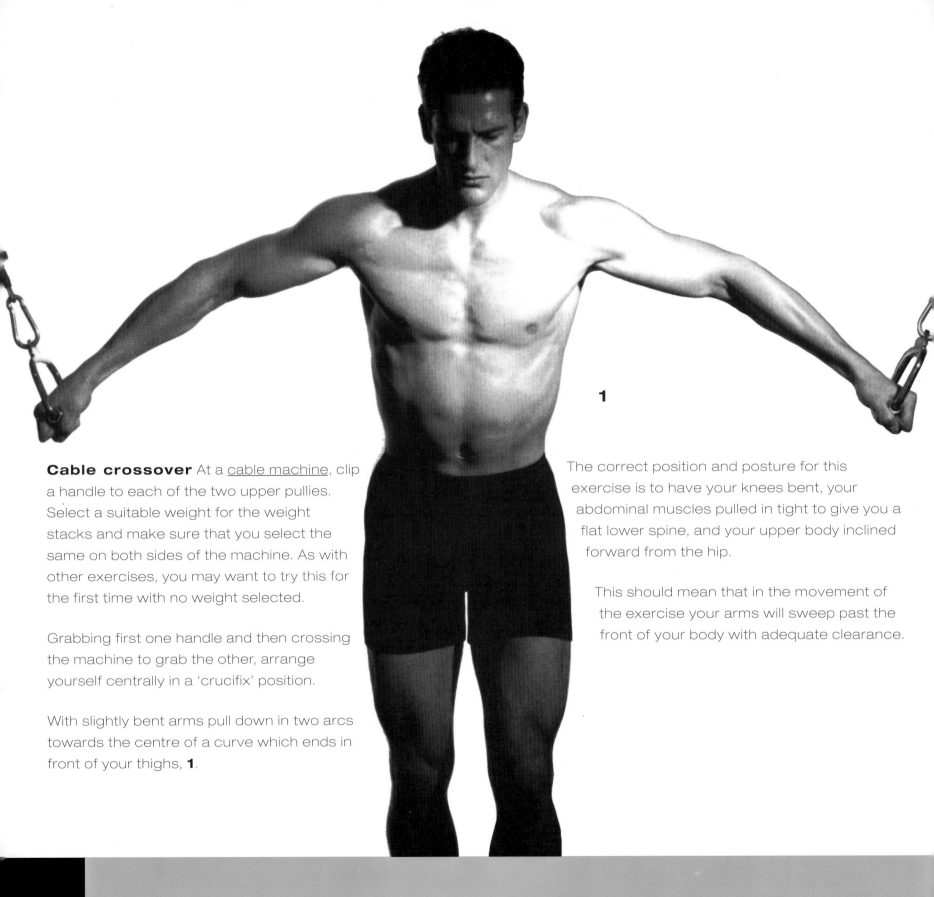

1

Cable crossover At a <u>cable machine</u>, clip a handle to each of the two upper pullies. Select a suitable weight for the weight stacks and make sure that you select the same on both sides of the machine. As with other exercises, you may want to try this for the first time with no weight selected.

Grabbing first one handle and then crossing the machine to grab the other, arrange yourself centrally in a 'crucifix' position.

With slightly bent arms pull down in two arcs towards the centre of a curve which ends in front of your thighs, **1**.

The correct position and posture for this exercise is to have your knees bent, your abdominal muscles pulled in tight to give you a flat lower spine, and your upper body inclined forward from the hip.

This should mean that in the movement of the exercise your arms will sweep past the front of your body with adequate clearance.

Continue to pull down, as if your hands are going to meet, **2**, with arms still slightly bent.

Moving one hand nearer to your body and the other farther away, continue the downward movement so that your hands cross over. There is a limit to how far you can go as your forearms will start to clash with the cables.

Control the movement back to the start of the 'crucifix', all the while keeping arms slightly bent.

Continue to exhaustion, crossing your hands over alternately in front and behind each other.

2

Return first one pulley to the resting position, then the other.

When crossing the cables over, take care to make sure you do not scrape the knuckles of one hand with the handle held by the other.

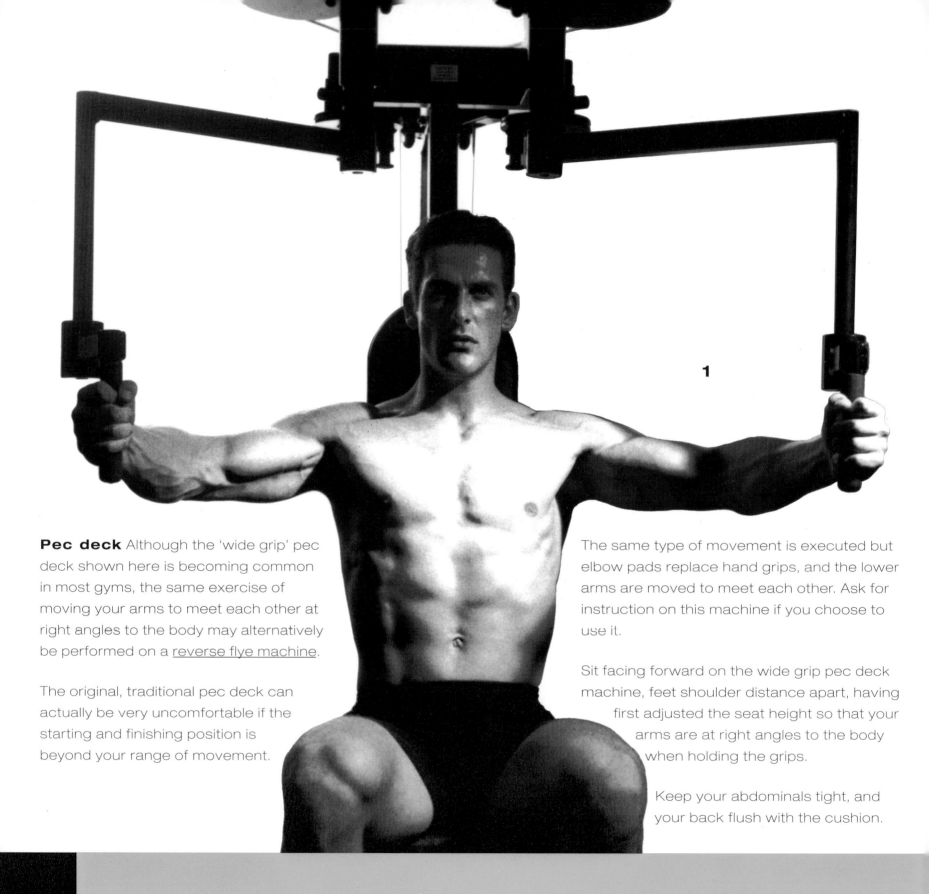

1

Pec deck Although the 'wide grip' pec deck shown here is becoming common in most gyms, the same exercise of moving your arms to meet each other at right angles to the body may alternatively be performed on a <u>reverse flye machine</u>.

The original, traditional pec deck can actually be very uncomfortable if the starting and finishing position is beyond your range of movement.

The same type of movement is executed but elbow pads replace hand grips, and the lower arms are moved to meet each other. Ask for instruction on this machine if you choose to use it.

Sit facing forward on the wide grip pec deck machine, feet shoulder distance apart, having first adjusted the seat height so that your arms are at right angles to the body when holding the grips.

Keep your abdominals tight, and your back flush with the cushion.

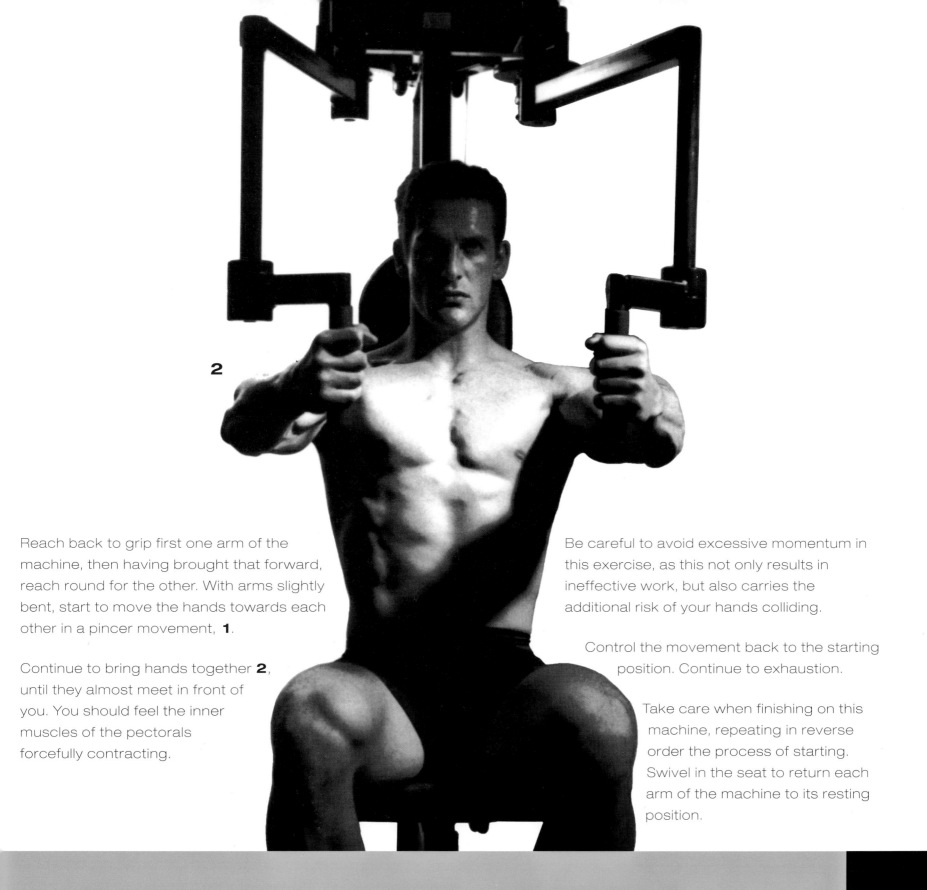

2

Reach back to grip first one arm of the machine, then having brought that forward, reach round for the other. With arms slightly bent, start to move the hands towards each other in a pincer movement, **1**.

Continue to bring hands together **2**, until they almost meet in front of you. You should feel the inner muscles of the pectorals forcefully contracting.

Be careful to avoid excessive momentum in this exercise, as this not only results in ineffective work, but also carries the additional risk of your hands colliding.

Control the movement back to the starting position. Continue to exhaustion.

Take care when finishing on this machine, repeating in reverse order the process of starting. Swivel in the seat to return each arm of the machine to its resting position.

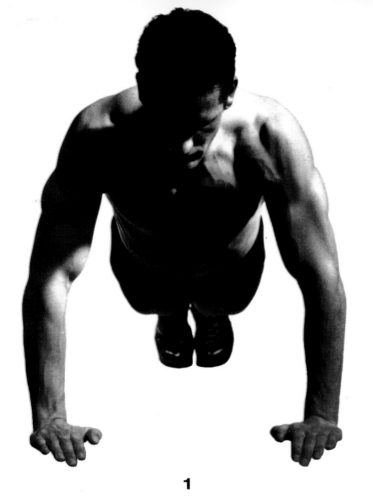

1

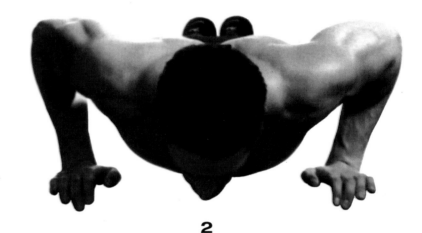

2

Press-up This simple but extremely effective exercise is eminently portable and can actually be performed anywhere with no equipment at all. So there is no excuse to exclude it from your chest routine, and the surroundings of the gym should help make sure you do not cheat, which is all too easily done.

Start by kneeling on the ground, then reach forward to place your hands slightly wider than shoulder distance apart on the ground in front of you. Walk back with your knees, working yourself on to your toes until head, back and legs are in one straight line, with no arching of the back, **1**.

Lower your body,controlling the downward movement with your arms in a smooth movement, going as low as you can without actually touching the ground, **2**, before raising to the starting position once more, arms almost straight.

Repeat to exhaustion.

Press-up variations Try some of these:

Incline press-up Standard, wide or close grip press-up technique, but your feet are on the ground and your hands on the edge of a bench. Works the upper pectorals.

Decline press-up Standard, wide or close grip press-up technique, but your feet are on a bench and your hands on the floor. Works the lower pectorals.

Wide grip press-up Much more difficult to do, the hands are positioned up to two shoulder widths apart, **1**, meaning the up and down movements are less, **2**, but the strength required to perform the movement is greater. This exercise stresses the lateral aspect of the pectoral muscles.

Close-grip press-up Even more difficult to do, and beyond the range of most, the hands are positioned only about a hands width apart. This is less effective as a chest exercise and actually mostly works the triceps muscles of the arms.

Press-up with stands You can do all of the standard and variation techniques using stands, which are almost like large cupboard handles on feet. They are less inclined to cause hand strain through the over-extension of joints than when performing regular press ups, provide a good grip on the floor, and extend the range of motion without the danger of hitting your nose on the floor. They appear to make push-ups easier, so be careful not to over-extend.

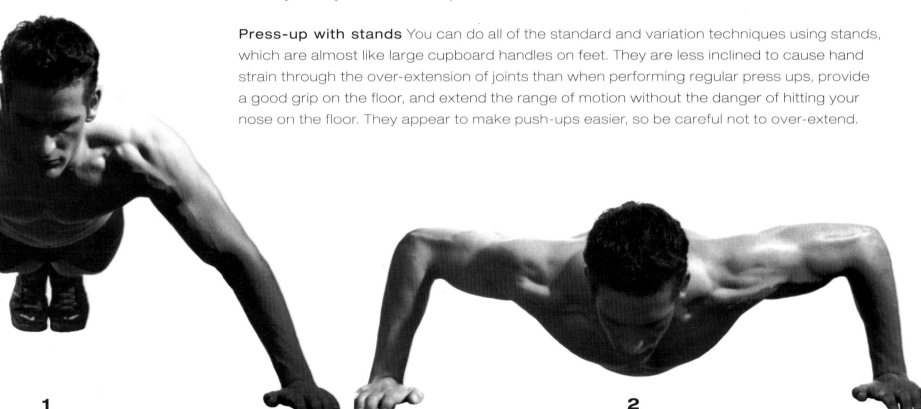

1

2

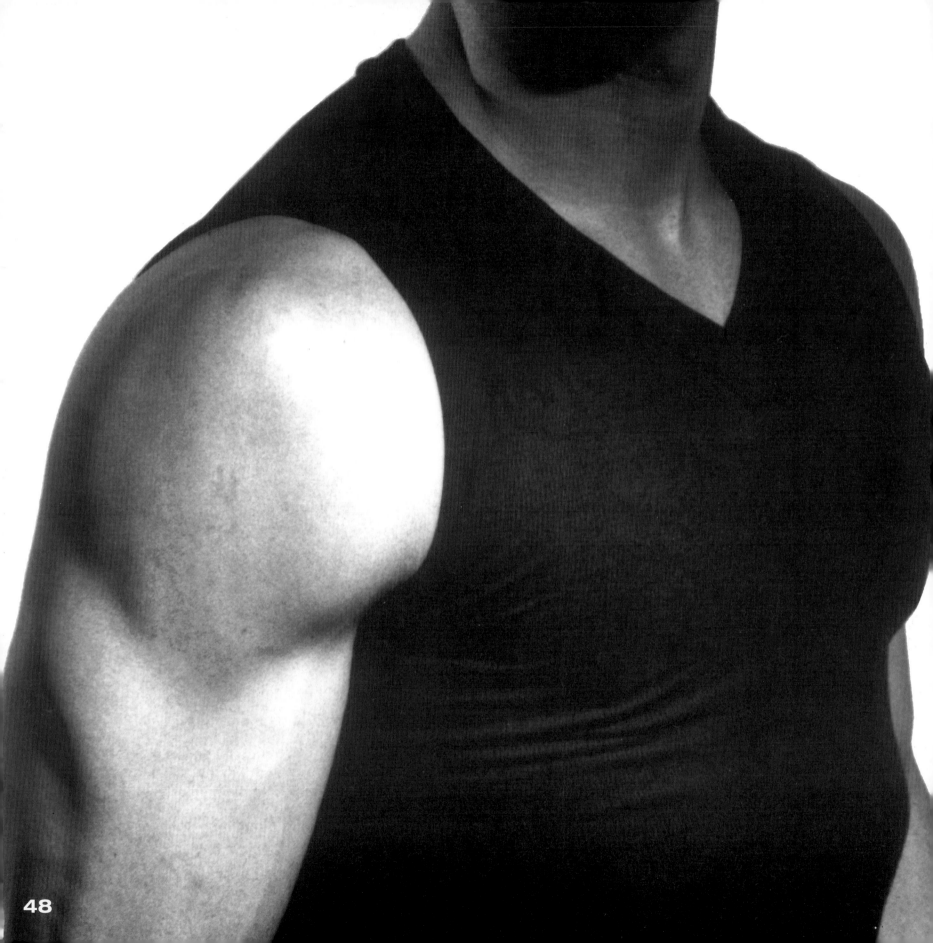

Broad shoulders have long been regarded as a symbol of strength, and the physical emphasis that well-shaped shoulders give to the torso make this hard-gained body part a much-desired goal.

SERVICING OF MOVING PARTS

SHOULDERS

The key component muscles are the **deltoids** (the rounded conclusion of the upper arm) and the **trapezius** muscles (the line running from neck to shoulder).

Section essentials

All exercises should be performed to exhaustion, i.e. to the point at which you cannot achieve another rep.

The weight selected should be chosen to achieve the following ratio of reps and sets for *either*

Endurance work:

2–3 sets of 15–20 reps

or

Muscle building work:

3–5 sets of 6–8 reps

Rest between sets for only the length of time it has taken you to perform the previous set.

Take a deep breath prior to starting an exercise, then exhale on the <u>exertion</u> and inhale on the <u>recovery</u>. Do not hold your breath – this may dangerously elevate the blood pressure.

Where your arms or legs are working towards being straight, take care not to '<u>lock out</u>'. Keep limbs slightly bent.

Explore possibilities beyond the exercises shown. Ask for instruction on <u>isolation machines</u> available for specific body parts that you can add into your programme for variety.

Military press Select a suitable barbell, then sit at an upright bench, which is actually like a chair. If your gym does not have one, your can set an incline bench upright, with the seat pad flat. Your hands should grip the barbell slightly wider than shoulder width, and your feet should be firmly on the floor, shoulder distance apart, abdominals in tight.

Raise the barbell to the start position at the top of your chest, **1**, **2**.

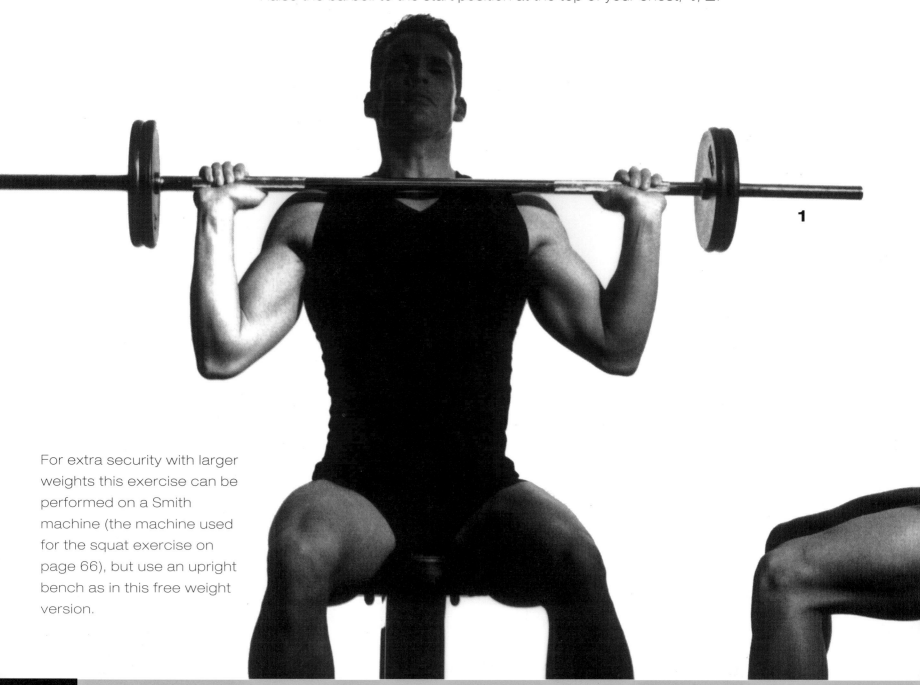

1

For extra security with larger weights this exercise can be performed on a Smith machine (the machine used for the squat exercise on page 66), but use an upright bench as in this free weight version.

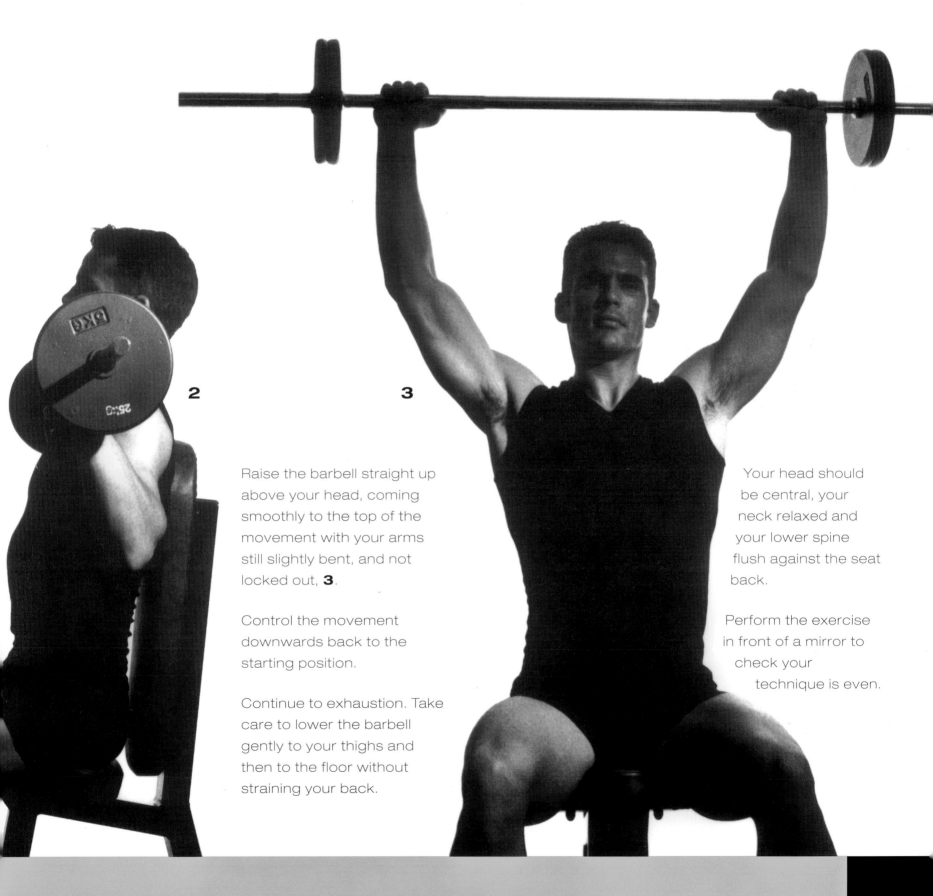

2

3

Raise the barbell straight up above your head, coming smoothly to the top of the movement with your arms still slightly bent, and not locked out, **3**.

Control the movement downwards back to the starting position.

Continue to exhaustion. Take care to lower the barbell gently to your thighs and then to the floor without straining your back.

Your head should be central, your neck relaxed and your lower spine flush against the seat back.

Perform the exercise in front of a mirror to check your technique is even.

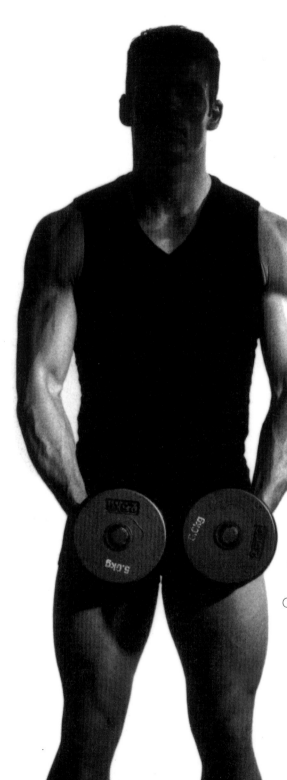

1

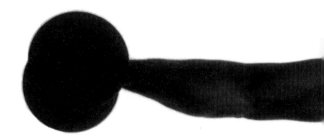

Lateral raise Only a very light weight is needed for this exercise to be effective, and for the first time you perform this exercise select the lightest pair of dumb-bells available. Learning correct technique for the lateral raise is very important, as it is one of the easiest exercises to get wrong.

Stand with your feet shoulder distance apart, knees slightly bent, stomach in tight, with the selected dumb-bells held in front of you and arms slightly bent, **1**. Doing this exercise in front of a mirror may help you to assess the quality of your technique.

Raise your arms out to your sides, keeping arms slightly bent, until your hands are just above your shoulder level, **2**.

Control the movement downwards to the starting postion. Continue to exhaustion.

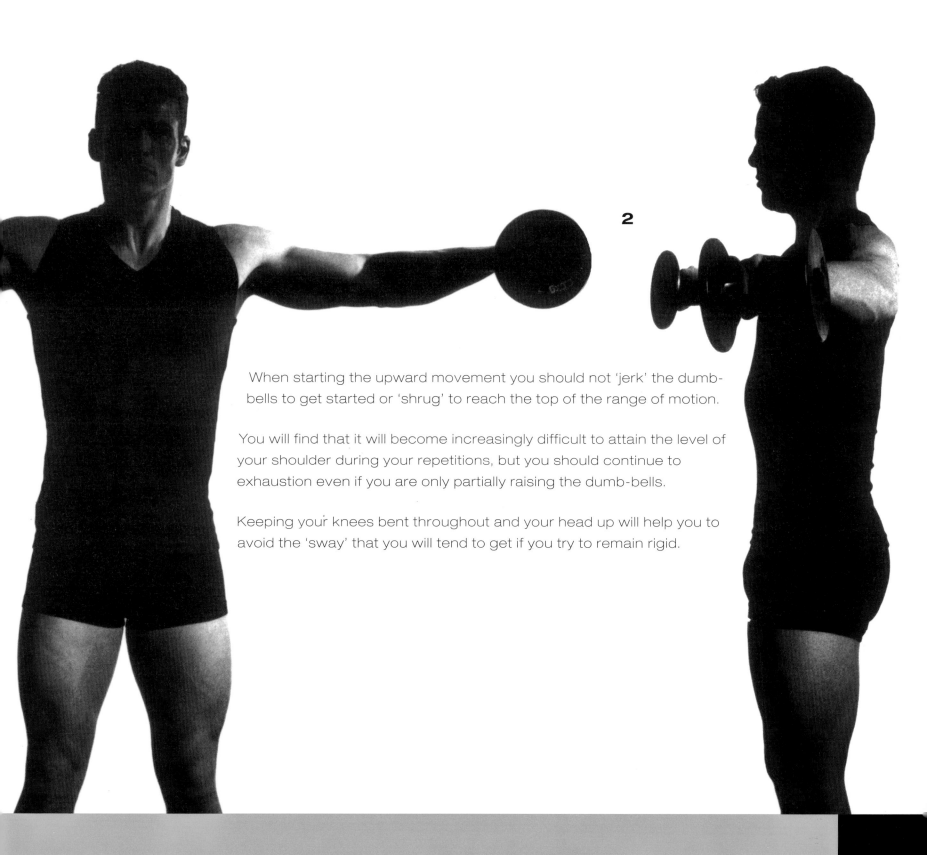

2

When starting the upward movement you should not 'jerk' the dumb-bells to get started or 'shrug' to reach the top of the range of motion.

You will find that it will become increasingly difficult to attain the level of your shoulder during your repetitions, but you should continue to exhaustion even if you are only partially raising the dumb-bells.

Keeping your knees bent throughout and your head up will help you to avoid the 'sway' that you will tend to get if you try to remain rigid.

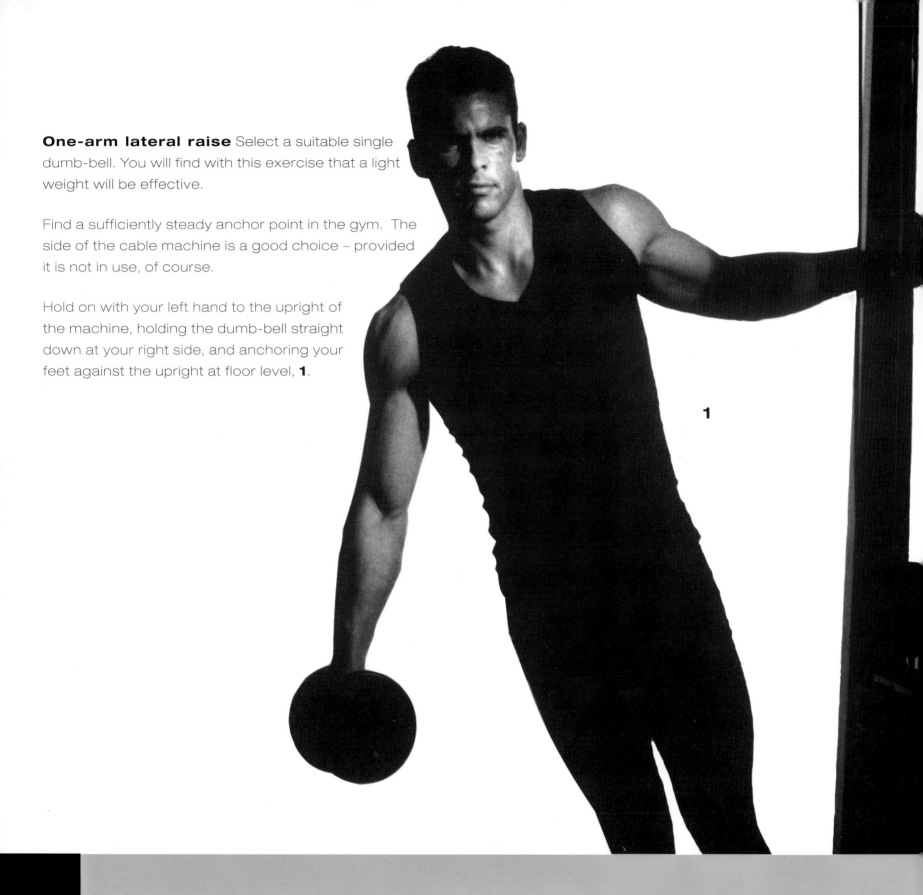

One-arm lateral raise Select a suitable single dumb-bell. You will find with this exercise that a light weight will be effective.

Find a sufficiently steady anchor point in the gym. The side of the cable machine is a good choice – provided it is not in use, of course.

Hold on with your left hand to the upright of the machine, holding the dumb-bell straight down at your right side, and anchoring your feet against the upright at floor level, **1**.

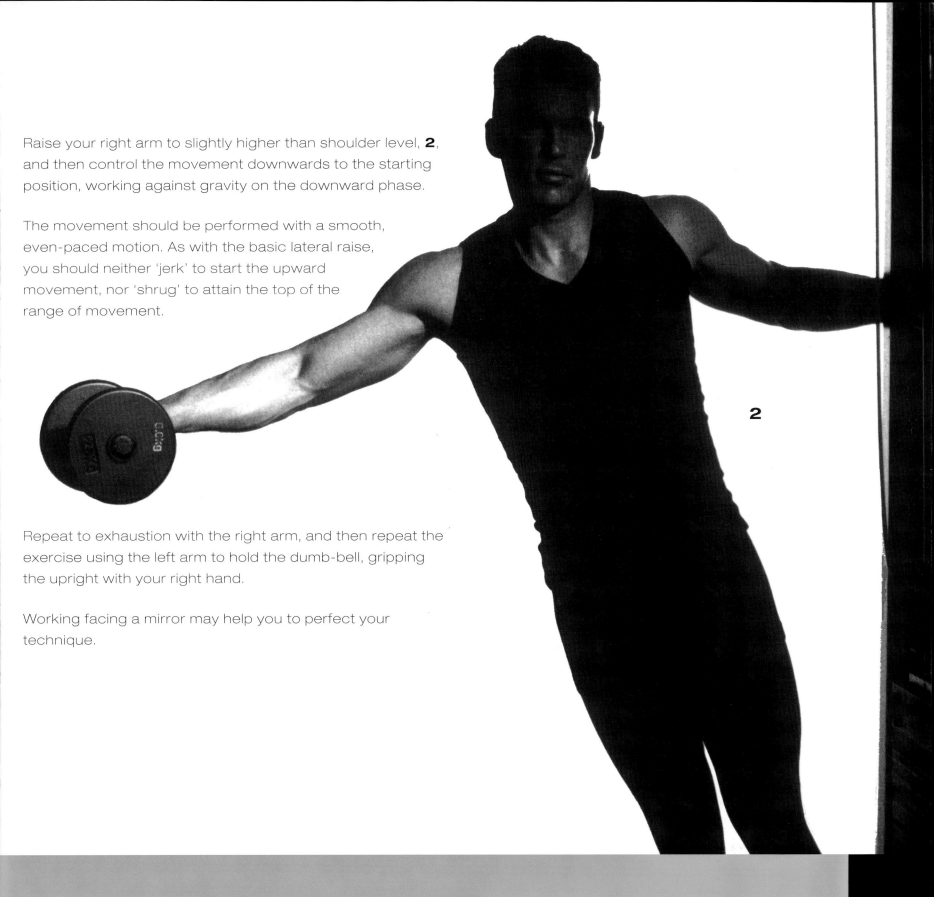

Raise your right arm to slightly higher than shoulder level, **2**, and then control the movement downwards to the starting position, working against gravity on the downward phase.

The movement should be performed with a smooth, even-paced motion. As with the basic lateral raise, you should neither 'jerk' to start the upward movement, nor 'shrug' to attain the top of the range of movement.

Repeat to exhaustion with the right arm, and then repeat the exercise using the left arm to hold the dumb-bell, gripping the upright with your right hand.

Working facing a mirror may help you to perfect your technique.

2

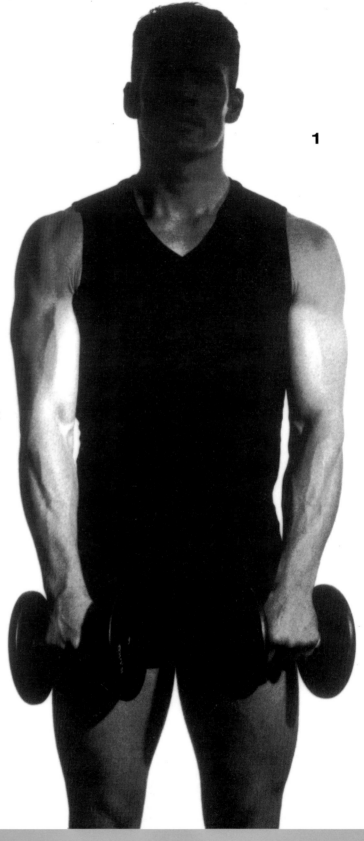

1

Front dumb-bell raise You should attempt higher weights than on the previous two exercises for this exercise, because it works the part of the deltoids that is usually strongest in most people.

Stand with the two selected dumb-bells hanging down in front of you with arms slightly bent, but try to avoid resting them against your thighs at the start and during the exercise. Stand with feet shoulder distance apart, legs slightly bent, **1**.

Keeping your knees bent throughout and your head up will help you to avoid the 'sway' that you will tend to get if you try to remain rigid.

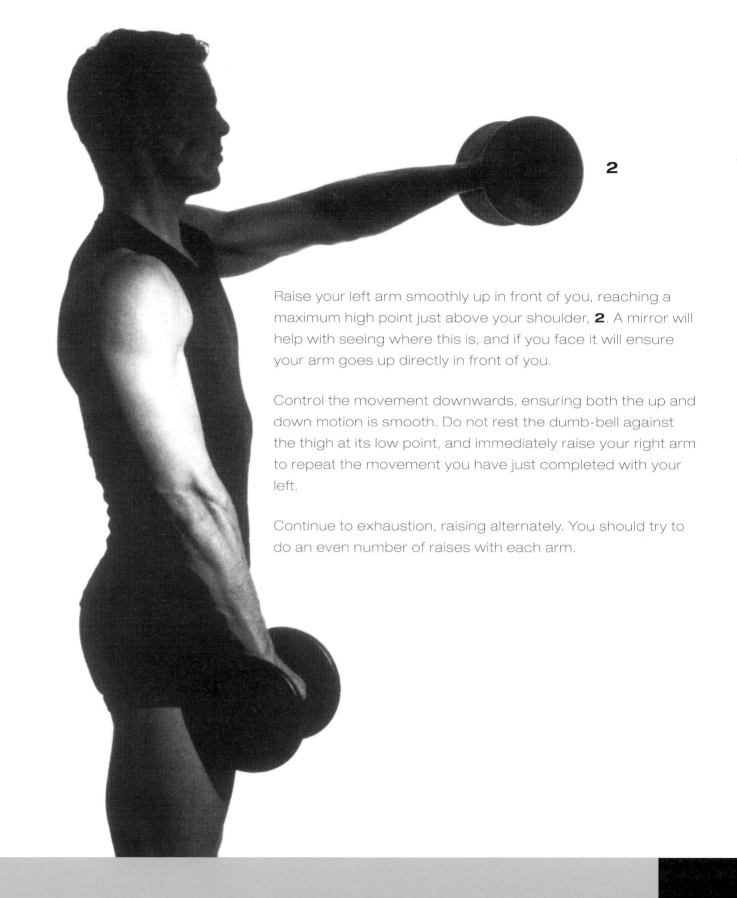

2

Raise your left arm smoothly up in front of you, reaching a maximum high point just above your shoulder, **2**. A mirror will help with seeing where this is, and if you face it will ensure your arm goes up directly in front of you.

Control the movement downwards, ensuring both the up and down motion is smooth. Do not rest the dumb-bell against the thigh at its low point, and immediately raise your right arm to repeat the movement you have just completed with your left.

Continue to exhaustion, raising alternately. You should try to do an even number of raises with each arm.

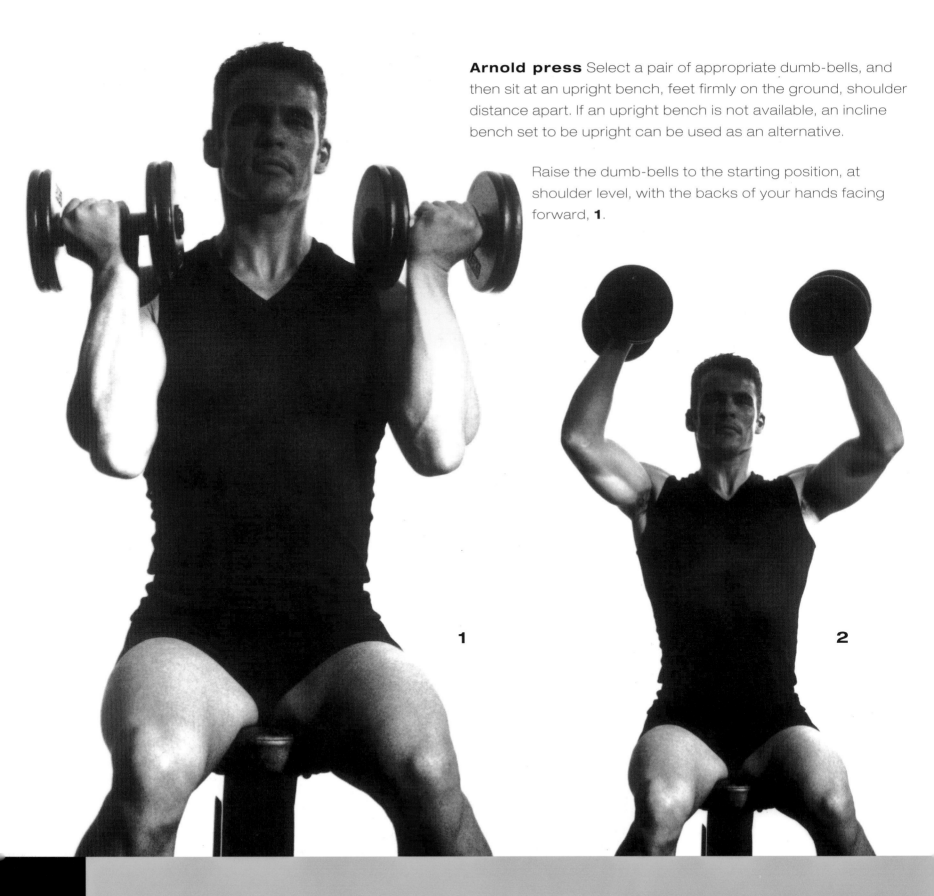

Arnold press Select a pair of appropriate dumb-bells, and then sit at an upright bench, feet firmly on the ground, shoulder distance apart. If an upright bench is not available, an incline bench set to be upright can be used as an alternative.

Raise the dumb-bells to the starting position, at shoulder level, with the backs of your hands facing forward, **1**.

1

2

Raise both arms at the same time from the starting position to a point at which each arm is fully extended over each corresponding shoulder, but do not lock out at the top of the movement.

As you raise the dumb-bells you need to rotate them, **2**, **3**, so that your hands finish with your palms facing forward, **4**.

This will take a little practice, so it may be a good idea to sit in front of a mirror and use very light weights to begin with.

Control the movement downwards, reversing the rotation so that you finish at the starting position again.

Continue to exhaustion.

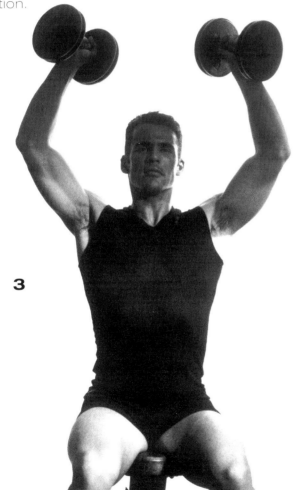

3

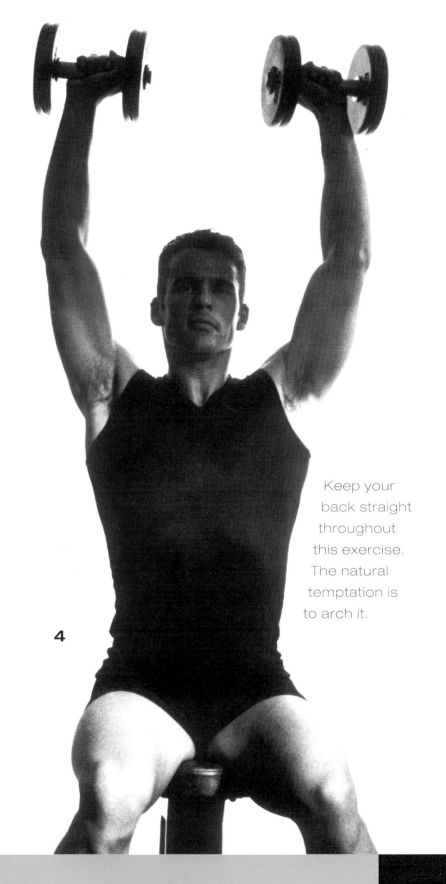

4

Keep your back straight throughout this exercise. The natural temptation is to arch it.

ARNOLD PRESS 59

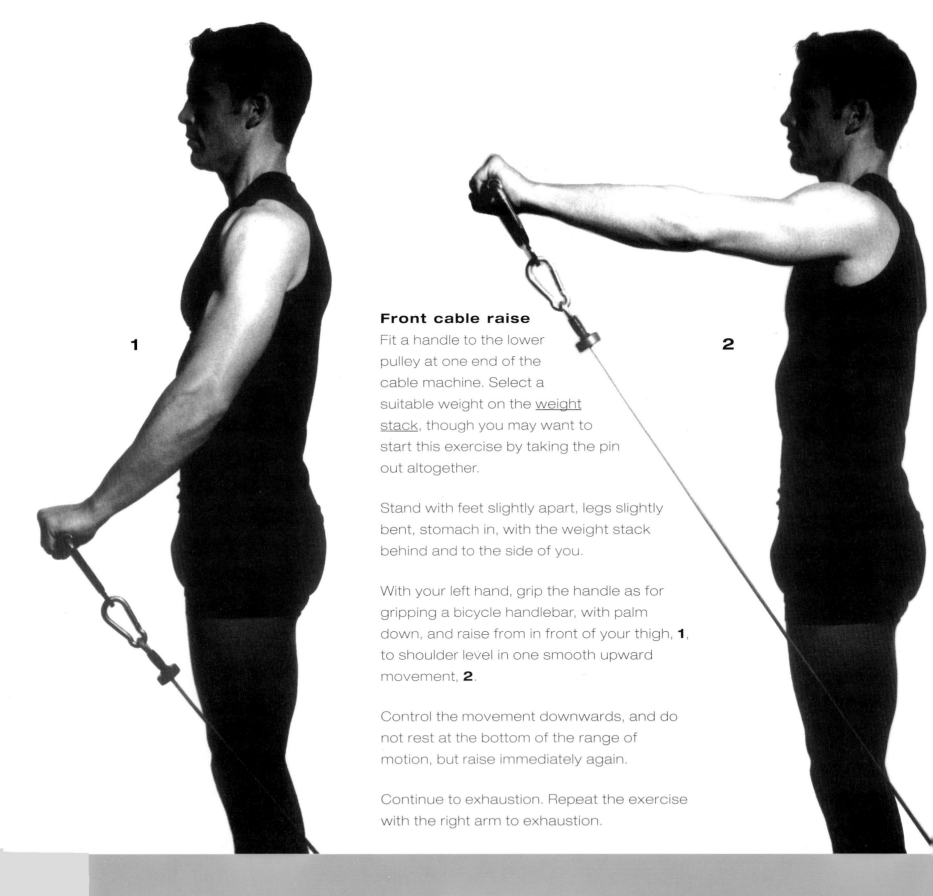

1

2

Front cable raise

Fit a handle to the lower
pulley at one end of the
cable machine. Select a
suitable weight on the <u>weight
stack</u>, though you may want to
start this exercise by taking the pin
out altogether.

Stand with feet slightly apart, legs slightly
bent, stomach in, with the weight stack
behind and to the side of you.

With your left hand, grip the handle as for
gripping a bicycle handlebar, with palm
down, and raise from in front of your thigh, **1**,
to shoulder level in one smooth upward
movement, **2**.

Control the movement downwards, and do
not rest at the bottom of the range of
motion, but raise immediately again.

Continue to exhaustion. Repeat the exercise
with the right arm to exhaustion.

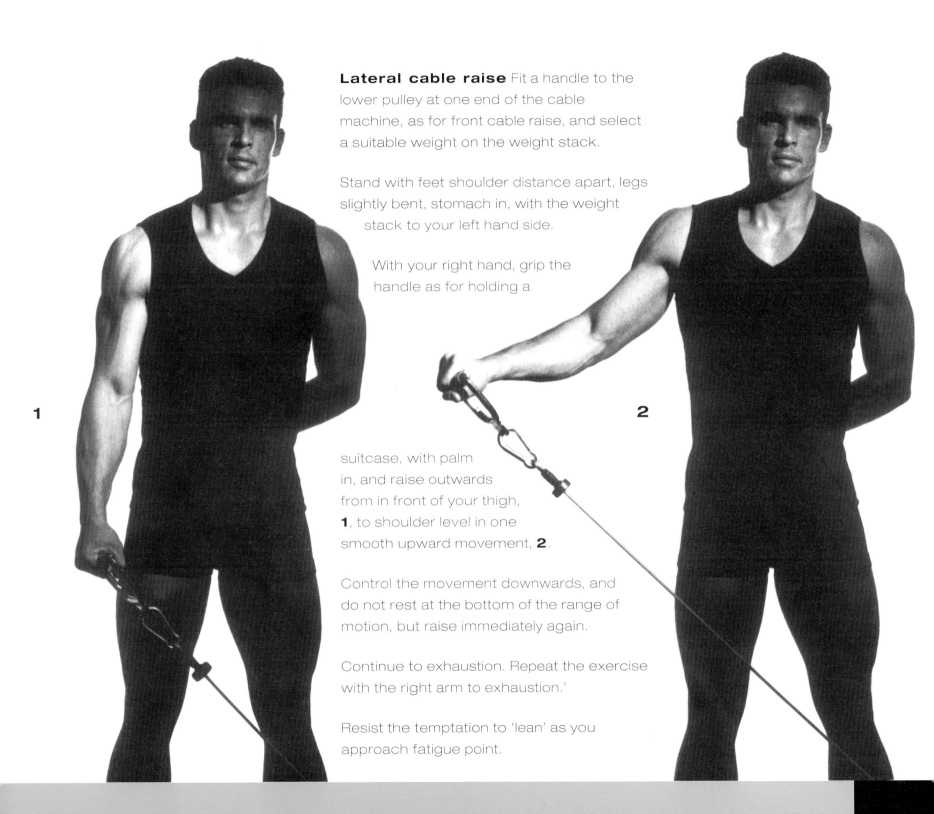

Lateral cable raise Fit a handle to the lower pulley at one end of the cable machine, as for front cable raise, and select a suitable weight on the weight stack.

Stand with feet shoulder distance apart, legs slightly bent, stomach in, with the weight stack to your left hand side.

With your right hand, grip the handle as for holding a

1

2

suitcase, with palm in, and raise outwards from in front of your thigh, **1**, to shoulder level in one smooth upward movement, **2**.

Control the movement downwards, and do not rest at the bottom of the range of motion, but raise immediately again.

Continue to exhaustion. Repeat the exercise with the right arm to exhaustion.'

Resist the temptation to 'lean' as you approach fatigue point.

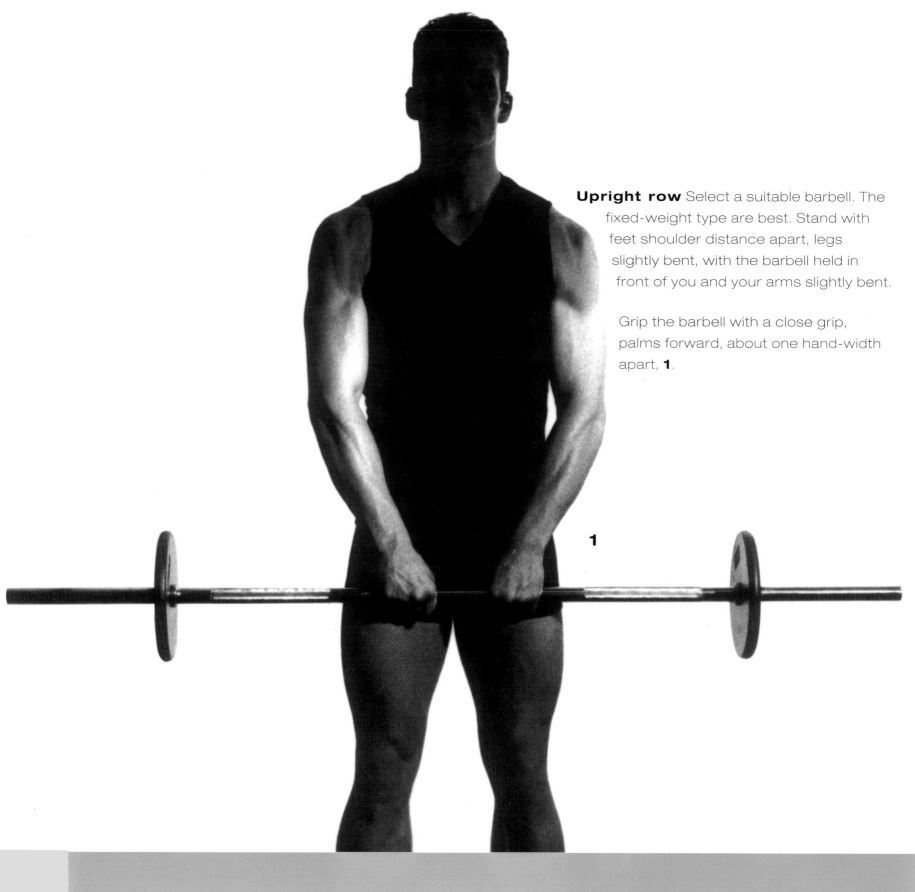

Upright row Select a suitable barbell. The fixed-weight type are best. Stand with feet shoulder distance apart, legs slightly bent, with the barbell held in front of you and your arms slightly bent.

Grip the barbell with a close grip, palms forward, about one hand-width apart, **1**.

1

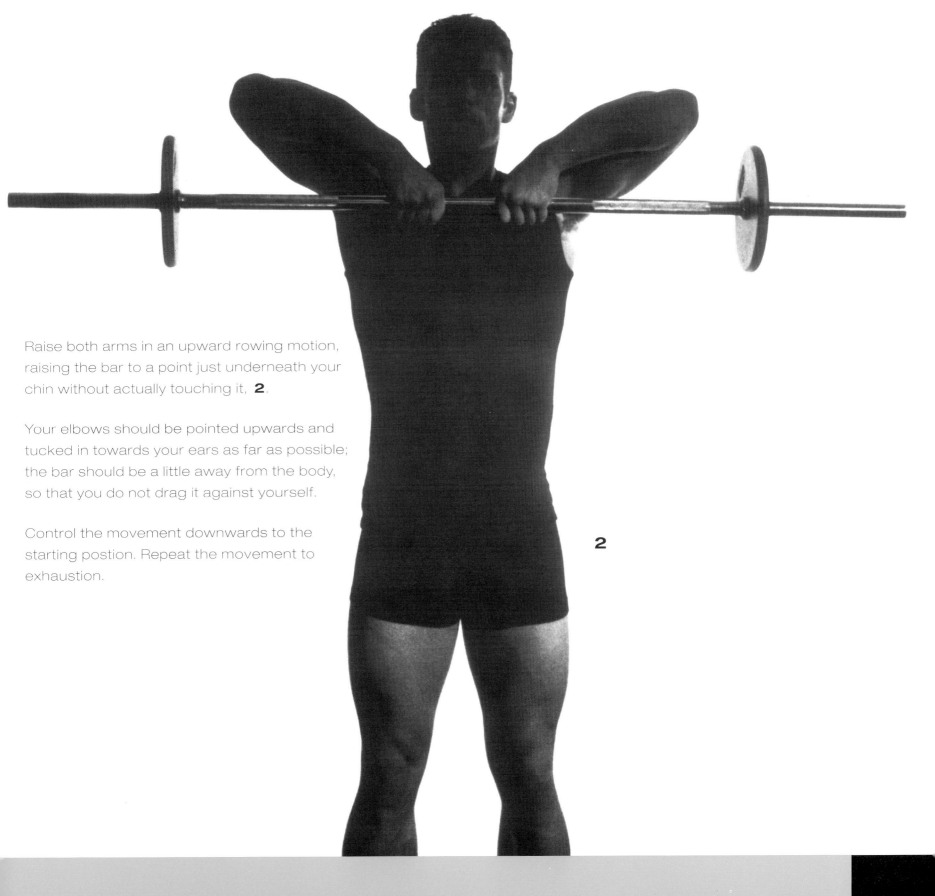

Raise both arms in an upward rowing motion, raising the bar to a point just underneath your chin without actually touching it, **2**.

Your elbows should be pointed upwards and tucked in towards your ears as far as possible; the bar should be a little away from the body, so that you do not drag it against yourself.

Control the movement downwards to the starting postion. Repeat the movement to exhaustion.

2

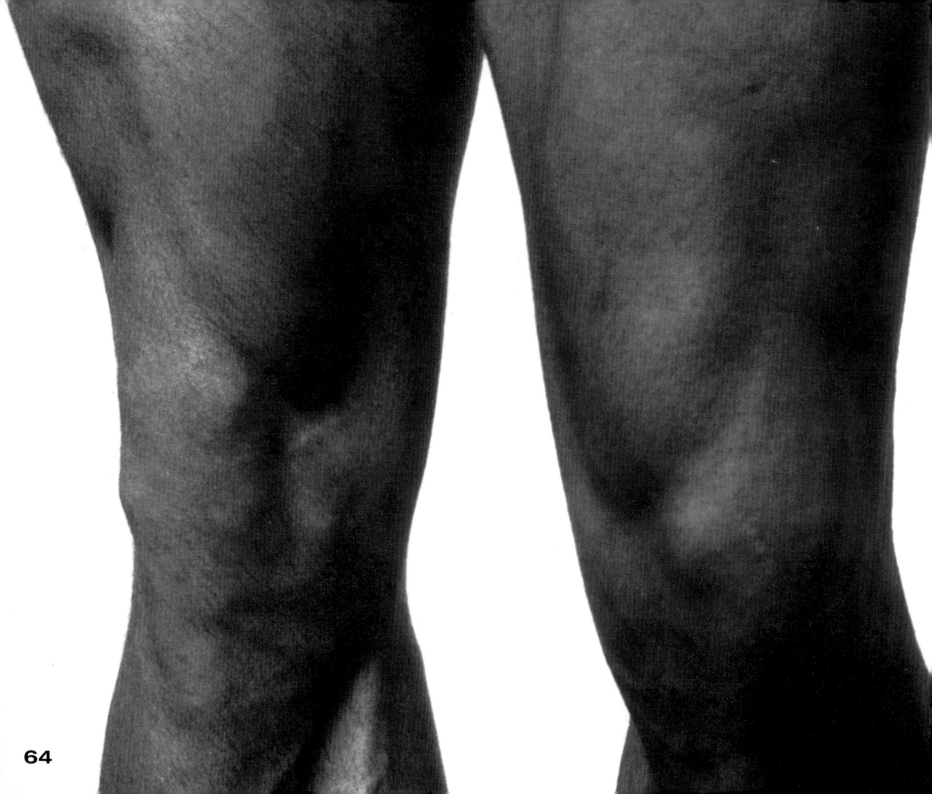

Curiously, the legs are the one part of the body men are usually more than happy to display – all year round. Crucial, then, that careful maintenance of these strong, visible body parts is diligently carried out.

SERVICING OF MOVING PARTS

LEGS

There are four major areas to be worked: **quads** (the front of the thigh) **hamstring** (the back of the upper leg) **gluteals** (the buttocks) and **calf** (the back of the lower leg).

Section essentials

All exercises should be performed to exhaustion, i.e. to the point at which you cannot achieve another rep.

The weight selected should be chosen to achieve the following ratio of reps and sets for *either*

Endurance work:
2–3 sets of 15–20 reps

or

Muscle building work:
3–5 sets of 6–8 reps

Rest between sets for only the length of time it has taken you to perform the previous set.

Take a deep breath prior to starting an exercise, then exhale on the exertion and inhale on the recovery. Do not hold your breath – this may dangerously elevate the blood pressure.

Where your legs are working towards being straight, take care not to 'lock out'. Keep limbs slightly bent.

Explore possibilities beyond the exercises shown. Ask for instruction on isolation machines available for specific body parts that you can add into your programme for variety.

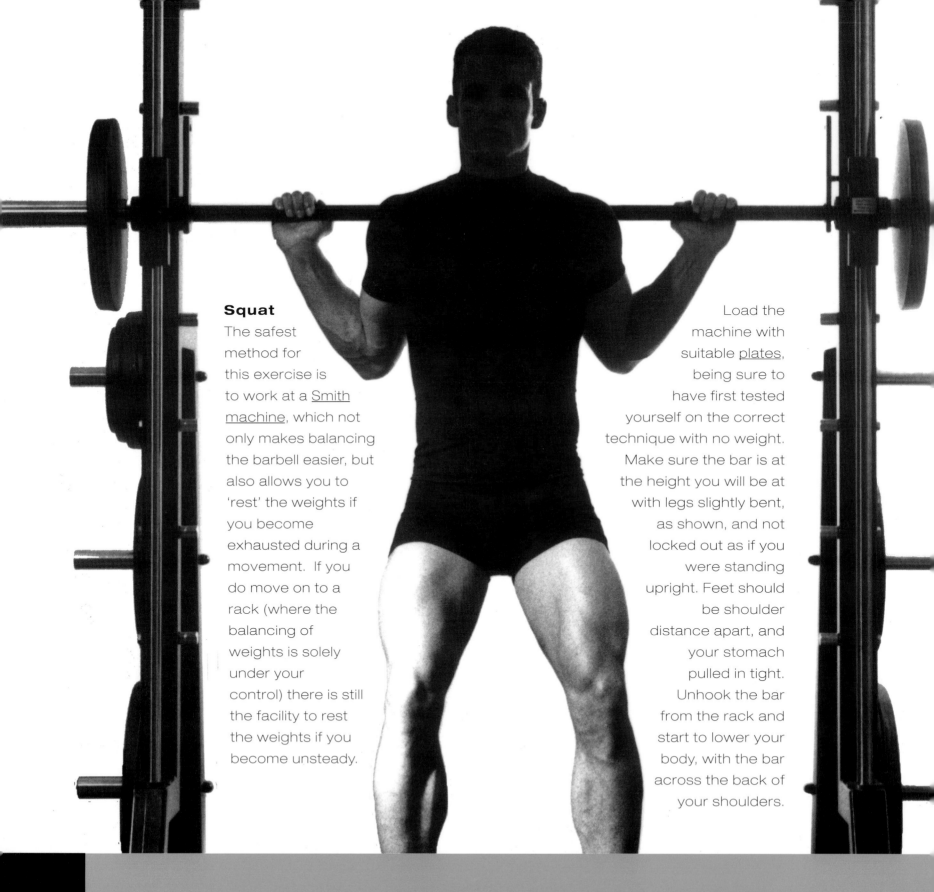

Squat

The safest method for this exercise is to work at a <u>Smith machine</u>, which not only makes balancing the barbell easier, but also allows you to 'rest' the weights if you become exhausted during a movement. If you do move on to a rack (where the balancing of weights is solely under your control) there is still the facility to rest the weights if you become unsteady.

Load the machine with suitable <u>plates</u>, being sure to have first tested yourself on the correct technique with no weight. Make sure the bar is at the height you will be at with legs slightly bent, as shown, and not locked out as if you were standing upright. Feet should be shoulder distance apart, and your stomach pulled in tight. Unhook the bar from the rack and start to lower your body, with the bar across the back of your shoulders.

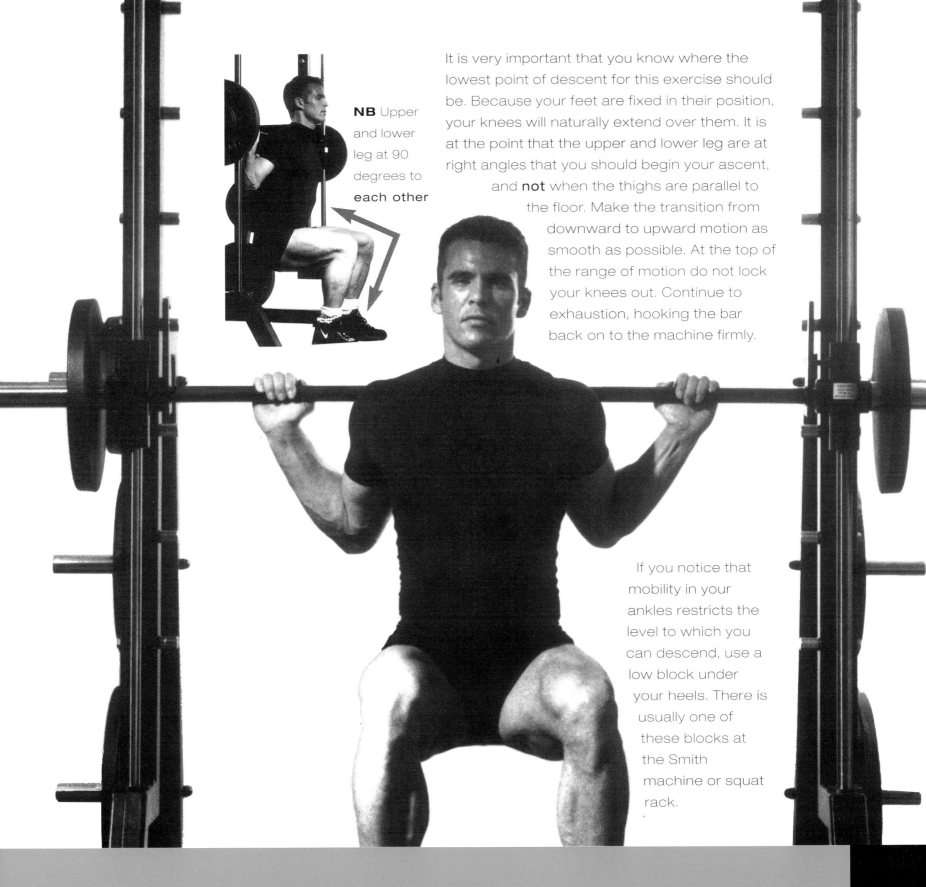

NB Upper and lower leg at 90 degrees to **each other**

It is very important that you know where the lowest point of descent for this exercise should be. Because your feet are fixed in their position, your knees will naturally extend over them. It is at the point that the upper and lower leg are at right angles that you should begin your ascent, and **not** when the thighs are parallel to the floor. Make the transition from downward to upward motion as smooth as possible. At the top of the range of motion do not lock your knees out. Continue to exhaustion, hooking the bar back on to the machine firmly.

If you notice that mobility in your ankles restricts the level to which you can descend, use a low block under your heels. There is usually one of these blocks at the Smith machine or squat rack.

SQUAT 67

Incline leg press You may be surprised at the amount of weight you can apply to this machine for your chosen number of reps, but because the exercise involves three out of the four strong muscle groups in the legs, the effort is shared.

Plates are loaded on the bars that stick out horizontally on the machine, and it is best to split the weight you are tackling in half between the two sides.

After first loading the machine, get into the seat, lie back and then lift your feet to place them on the platform that carries the weights. There are usually friction grip areas on the platform to show you how your feet should be positioned, ideally hip width apart.

Take the strain of the weight and ease slightly upwards with your legs, which will allow you to flick the locking handles out to the sides, **1**. These, when engaged, mean the weights cannot travel down beyond a certain point, but to do the exercise through the entire range of motion they will need to be disengaged.

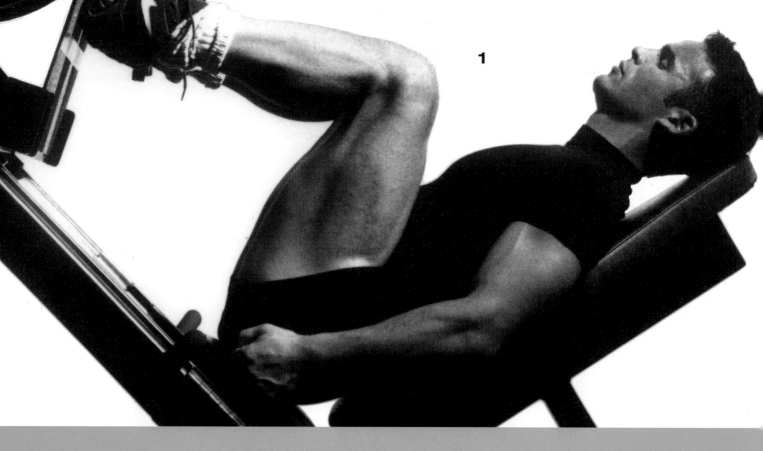

1

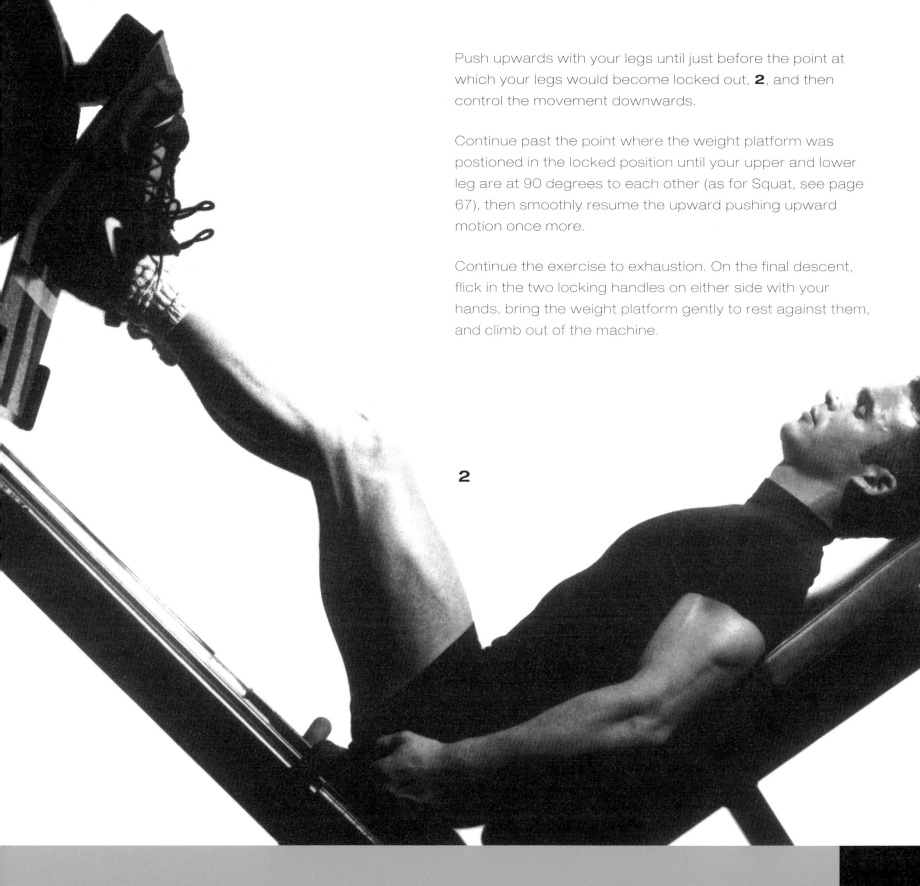

Push upwards with your legs until just before the point at which your legs would become locked out, **2**, and then control the movement downwards.

Continue past the point where the weight platform was postioned in the locked position until your upper and lower leg are at 90 degrees to each other (as for Squat, see page 67), then smoothly resume the upward pushing upward motion once more.

Continue the exercise to exhaustion. On the final descent, flick in the two locking handles on either side with your hands, bring the weight platform gently to rest against them, and climb out of the machine.

2

INCLINE LEG PRESS

Lunge and standing lunge The technique for both of these exercises is the same, the crucial difference being what you use to add the weight resistance. The lunge utilises a barbell held across the shoulders, **1**, the standing lunge a pair of dumb-bells held at the sides of the body, **2**. The standing lunge is easiest for the beginner because balance is easier to maintain.

From the standing position, for both exercises step one pace forward with either leg, and then take the knee of the rear leg towards the ground, **3**, but do not touch down. Reverse the step to regain the standing position. Repeat the movement with the other leg. Continue to exhaustion.

1

2

3

Keep your back up straight, by keeping your abs in tight.

Leading upper and lower leg should not go to less than 90 degrees.

Rear foot should be on its ball; there should be no twist at ankle or knee.

Feet should be as if on railway lines.

Alternate the legs.

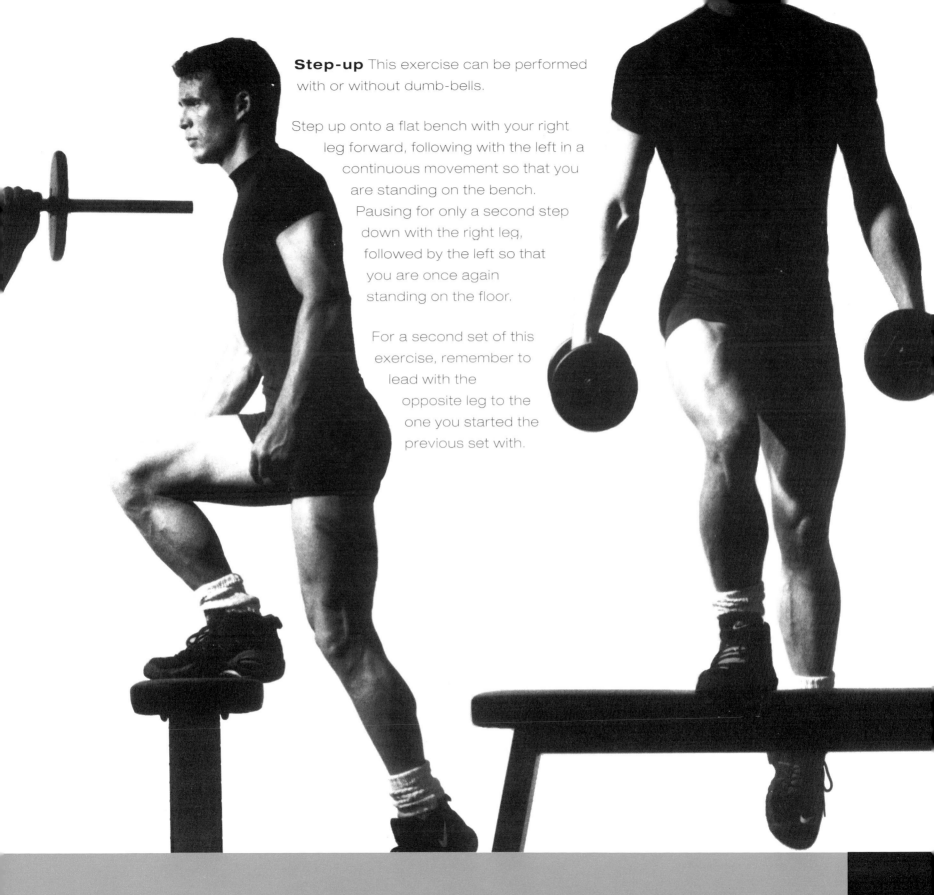

Step-up This exercise can be performed with or without dumb-bells.

Step up onto a flat bench with your right leg forward, following with the left in a continuous movement so that you are standing on the bench. Pausing for only a second step down with the right leg, followed by the left so that you are once again standing on the floor.

For a second set of this exercise, remember to lead with the opposite leg to the one you started the previous set with.

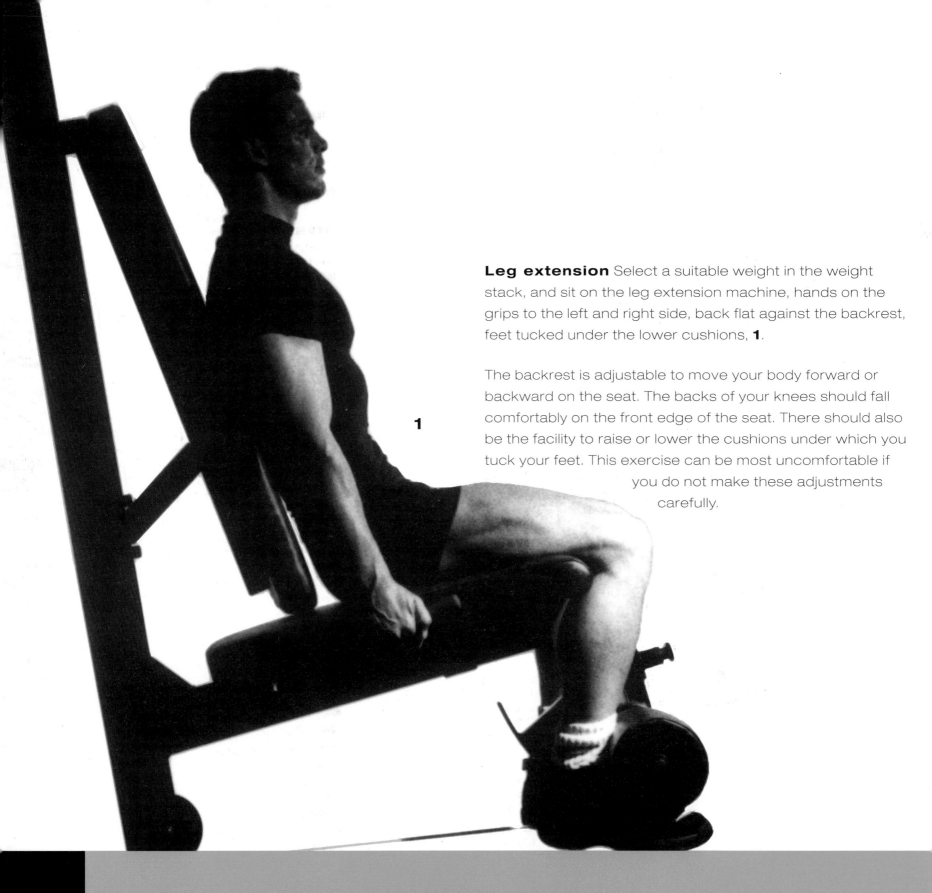

Leg extension Select a suitable weight in the weight stack, and sit on the leg extension machine, hands on the grips to the left and right side, back flat against the backrest, feet tucked under the lower cushions, **1**.

The backrest is adjustable to move your body forward or backward on the seat. The backs of your knees should fall comfortably on the front edge of the seat. There should also be the facility to raise or lower the cushions under which you tuck your feet. This exercise can be most uncomfortable if you do not make these adjustments carefully.

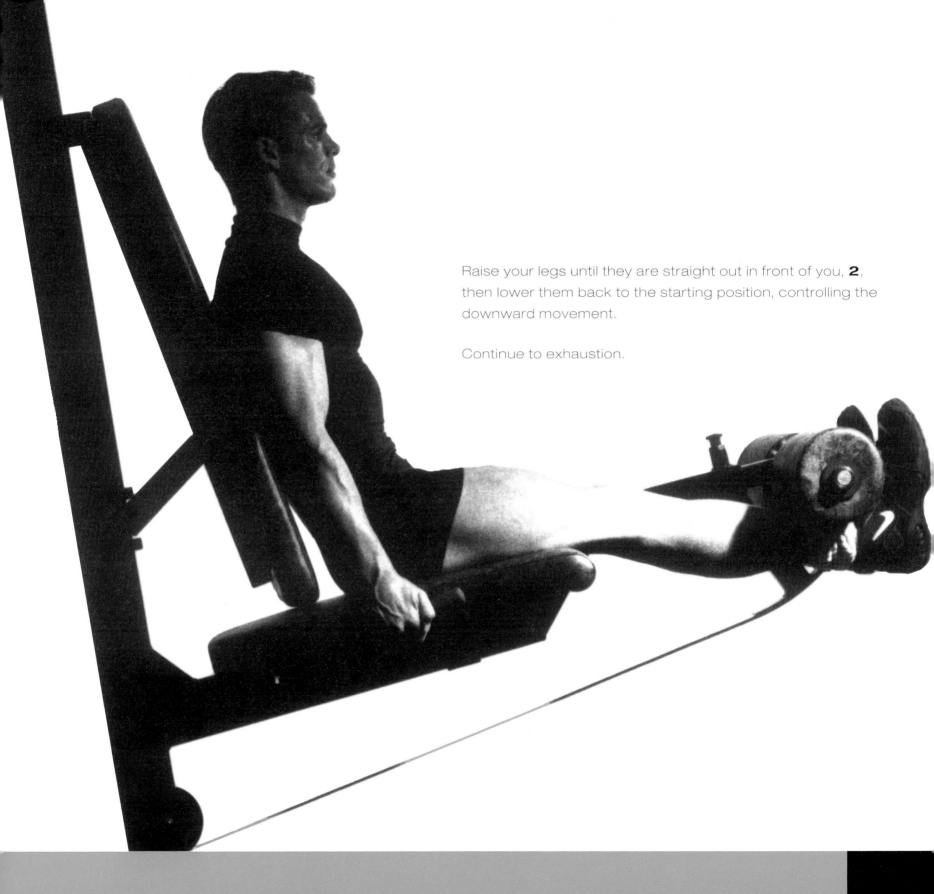

Raise your legs until they are straight out in front of you, **2**, then lower them back to the starting position, controlling the downward movement.

Continue to exhaustion.

Leg curl Select a suitable weight on the weight stack, then lie face down on the machine, tucking your heels under the cushions at the end of the arm which you will raise with your legs, **1**. The postion of this cushion is adjustable, and should be set so that it will not finish too low down your leg in the raised position, causing discomfort in the Achilles region.

Grasp the hand grips under the front of the machine, and then raise your legs, as if to press your heels against your buttocks, **2**. Work the movement to the fullest range you can – the adjusting knob should go between your legs.

Control the movement back to the starting position, then continue the exercise to exhaustion.

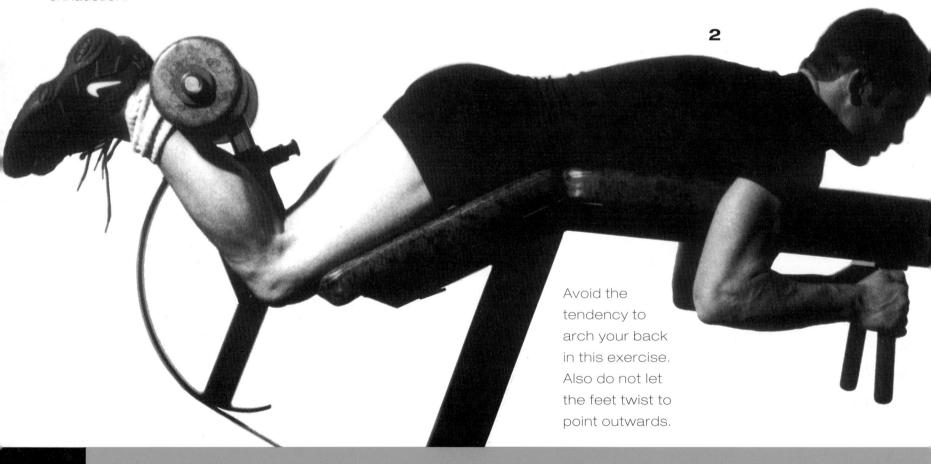

Avoid the tendency to arch your back in this exercise. Also do not let the feet twist to point outwards.

Standing leg curl Essentially performing the same movement as the leg curl, the standing leg curl differs in that it works one leg at a time.

Select a suitable weight on the weight stack. Stand on the left side of the machine, with your right hand holding the grip at the top of the machine to balance yourself. Hook your right foot behind the cushion at the base of the armature, **1**.

Raise your right leg in an attempt to bring your right heel to your right buttock, though you should stop short of this in practice. Control the movement downwards to the starting position.

Continue to exhaustion.

Change to the right side of the machine, and repeat the exercise to exhaustion with the left leg.

Avoid the tendency to arch your back in this exercise too.

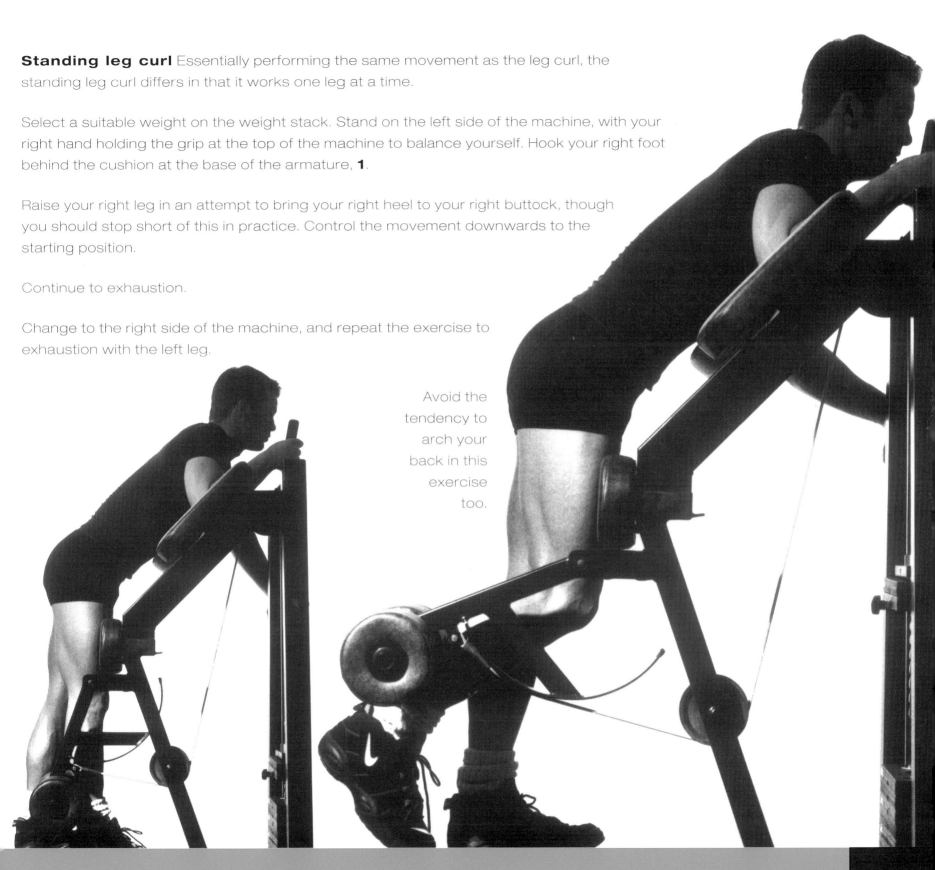

Seated leg curl Select a suitable weight on the weight stack. Sit at the machine, resting the backs of your lower calves on the cushion at the end of the armature. Adjust the position of this if necessary.

Adjust the leg clamp (the other cushion suspended over your lower thighs just above your knees) so that it is touching your leg, **1**. On some machines this is replaced by a cushion on a circular ratchet that locks over onto your leg.

Draw your legs back and down as far as is comfortable, **2**. Control the movement back to the starting position.

Continue to exhaustion.

Release the leg clamp cushion before getting off the machine.

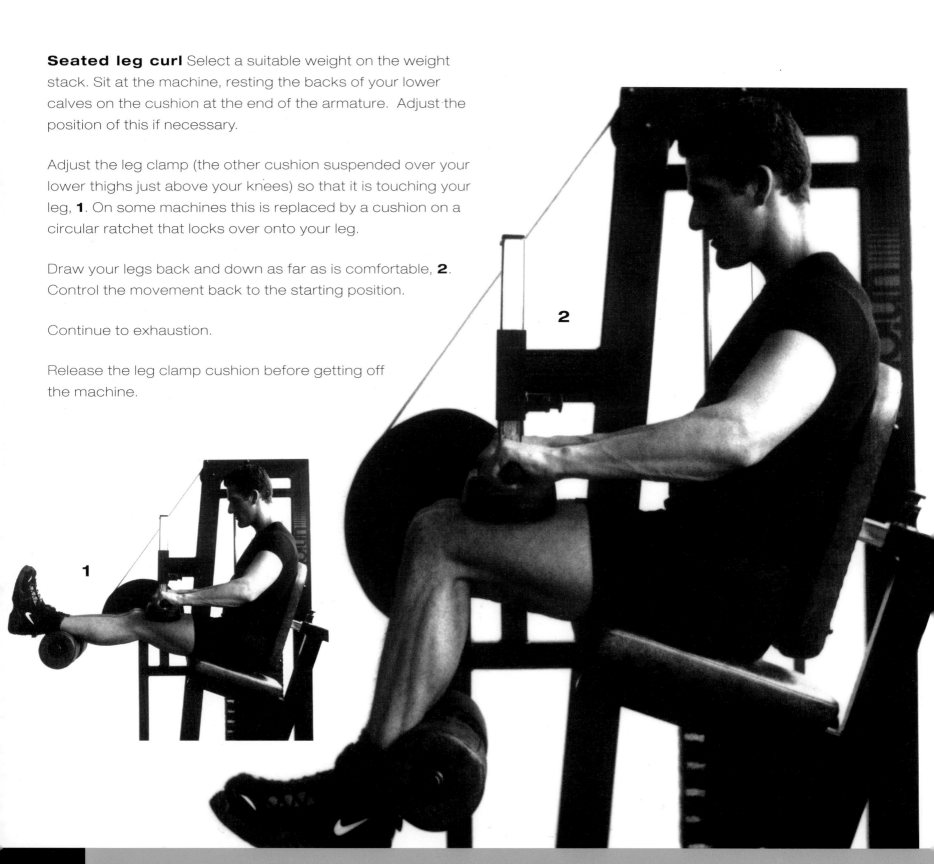

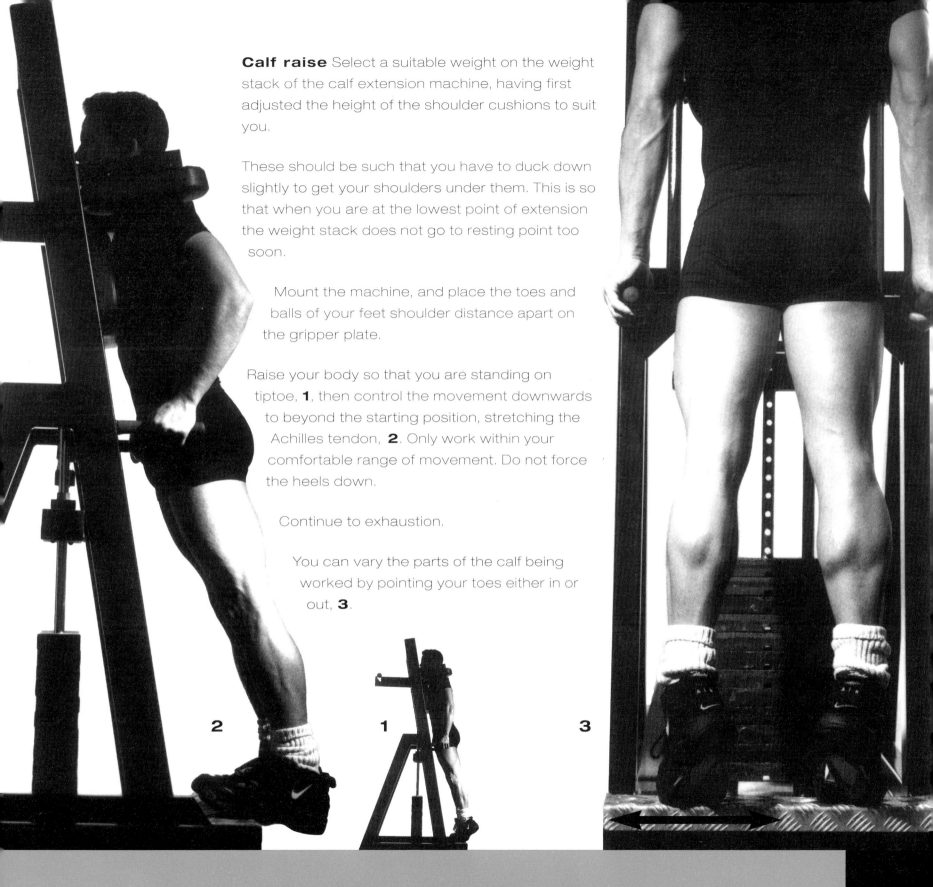

Calf raise Select a suitable weight on the weight stack of the calf extension machine, having first adjusted the height of the shoulder cushions to suit you.

These should be such that you have to duck down slightly to get your shoulders under them. This is so that when you are at the lowest point of extension the weight stack does not go to resting point too soon.

Mount the machine, and place the toes and balls of your feet shoulder distance apart on the gripper plate.

Raise your body so that you are standing on tiptoe, **1**, then control the movement downwards to beyond the starting position, stretching the Achilles tendon, **2**. Only work within your comfortable range of movement. Do not force the heels down.

Continue to exhaustion.

You can vary the parts of the calf being worked by pointing your toes either in or out, **3**.

2

1

3

Incline calf extension This machine needs to be loaded with plates. An equal weight should be applied to each side of the machine to maintain stability.

You will need to adjust the seat pad so that when you get into the machine your legs are slightly bent, otherwise the natural stopping position will mean that the lower point of the exercise cannot be reached.

Sit on the machine, holding on to the hand grips, and place your feet a little distance apart on the gripper plate, with only toes and balls of feet on the plate.

Straighten your legs, but trying not to fully lock out, and lower your heels below the gripper plate level, extending the Achilles tendon, **1**.

Raise your body by pointing your toes to go to tiptoe position, **2**, and then control the movement to the lower extension point once more.

Continue to exhaustion.

Variations to work different areas of the calf are an option, **3**, **4**.

1

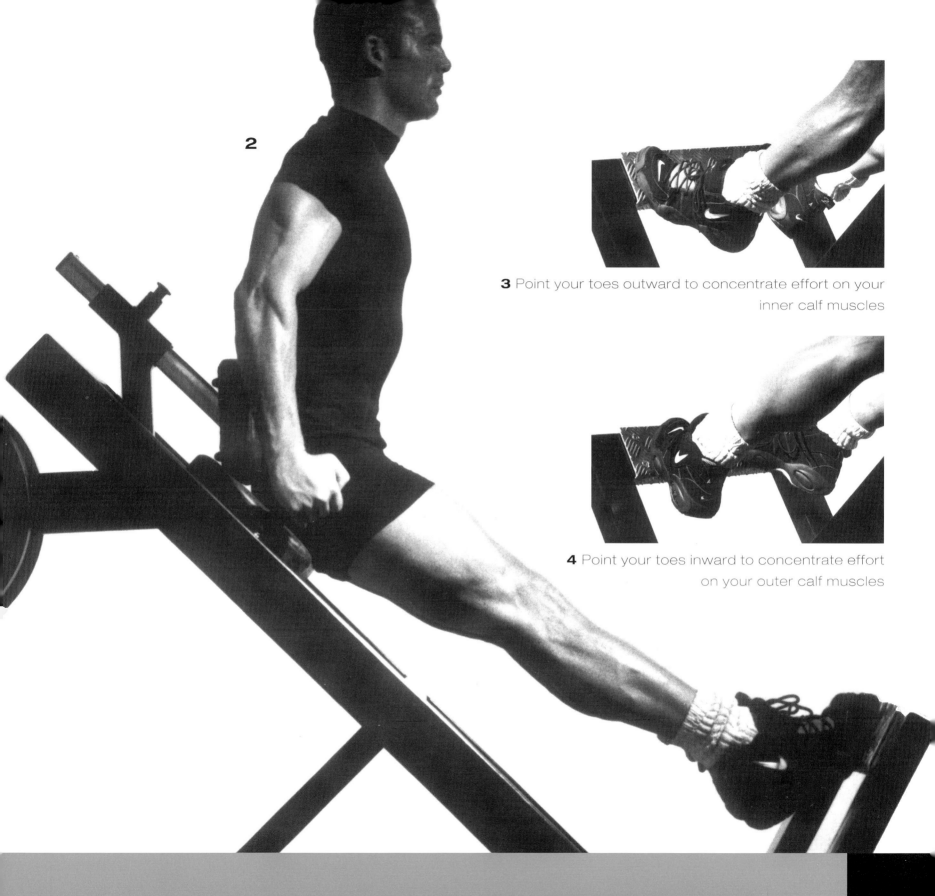

2

3 Point your toes outward to concentrate effort on your inner calf muscles

4 Point your toes inward to concentrate effort on your outer calf muscles

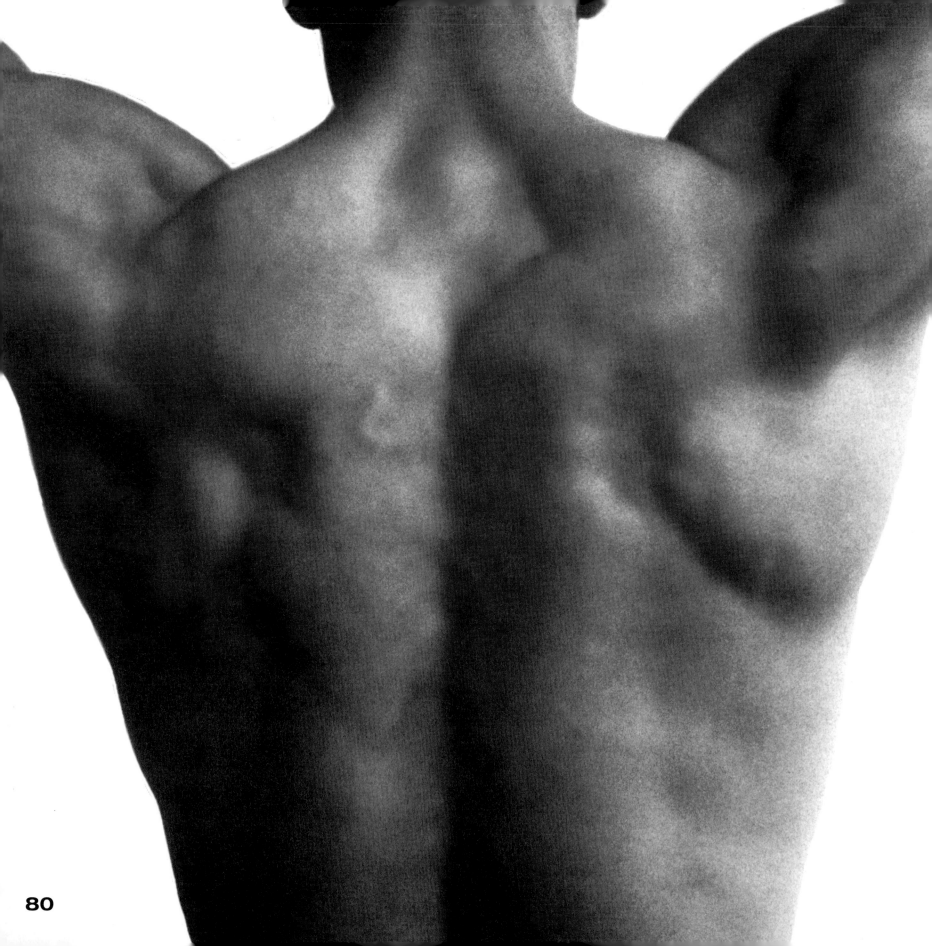

A classic 'V' physique should be the goal of any man keen to look his best. The area of the body that most contributes to the attainment of this shape is the upper back, which by its very nature will be more admired by others than by yourself.

SERVICING OF MOVING PARTS

BACK

The back is made up of many muscle groups, linked to form this strong and complex body part. Conversely, the lower back, the danger point for those with back problems, is also found here.

Section essentials

All exercises should be performed to exhaustion, i.e. to the point at which you cannot achieve another rep.

The weight selected should be chosen to achieve the following ratio of reps and sets for *either*

Endurance work:
2–3 sets of 15–20 reps

or

Muscle building work:
3–5 sets of 6–8 reps

Rest between sets for only the length of time it has taken you to perform the previous set.

Take a deep breath prior to starting an exercise, then exhale on the exertion and inhale on the recovery. Do not hold your breath – this may dangerously elevate the blood pressure.

Where your arms or legs are working towards being straight, take care not to 'lock out'. Keep limbs slightly bent.

Explore possibilities beyond the exercises shown. Ask for instruction on isolation machines available for specific body parts that you can add into your programme for variety.

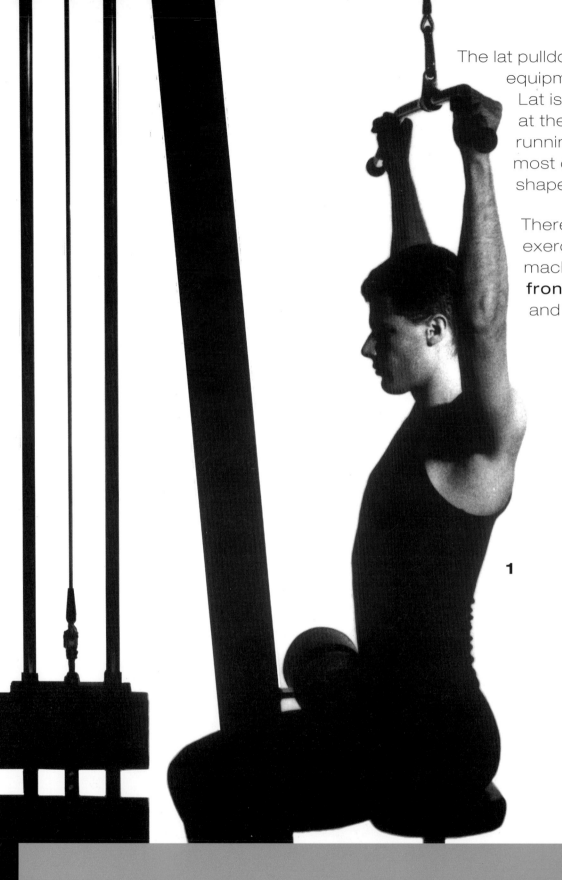

The lat pulldown machine is the key piece of equipment for working the upper back. Lat is short for *latissimus*, the muscle at the top of your back on each side, running from shoulder to waist, that most contributes to the classic 'V' shaped back.

There are three distinctly different exercises for the back on this machine: **wide grip pulldown to front**, **wide grip pulldown to rear**, and **close grip pulldown**.

1

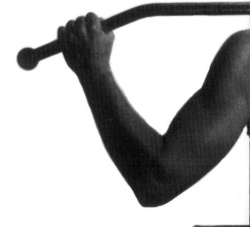

Don't get into the habit of relying on the touch of the bar behind your neck – if you get tired you may actually cause some damage to the top of your spine by striking it with the bar too firmly.

Wide grip pulldown to rear Clip the wide handle to the pulley of the lat pulldown machine, and then select a suitable weight on the weight stack. Adjust the seat height so that your thighs are tucked comfortably but firmly under the cushions. As most people cannot actually reach up to the bar once seated, the knack is to grasp the opposite ends of the bar with both hands, and then sit at the machine, **1**.

Pull the bar down, without jerking, so that it almost touches the top of your spine, **2**, **3**, and then control the movement back to the starting position.

Continue to exhaustion.

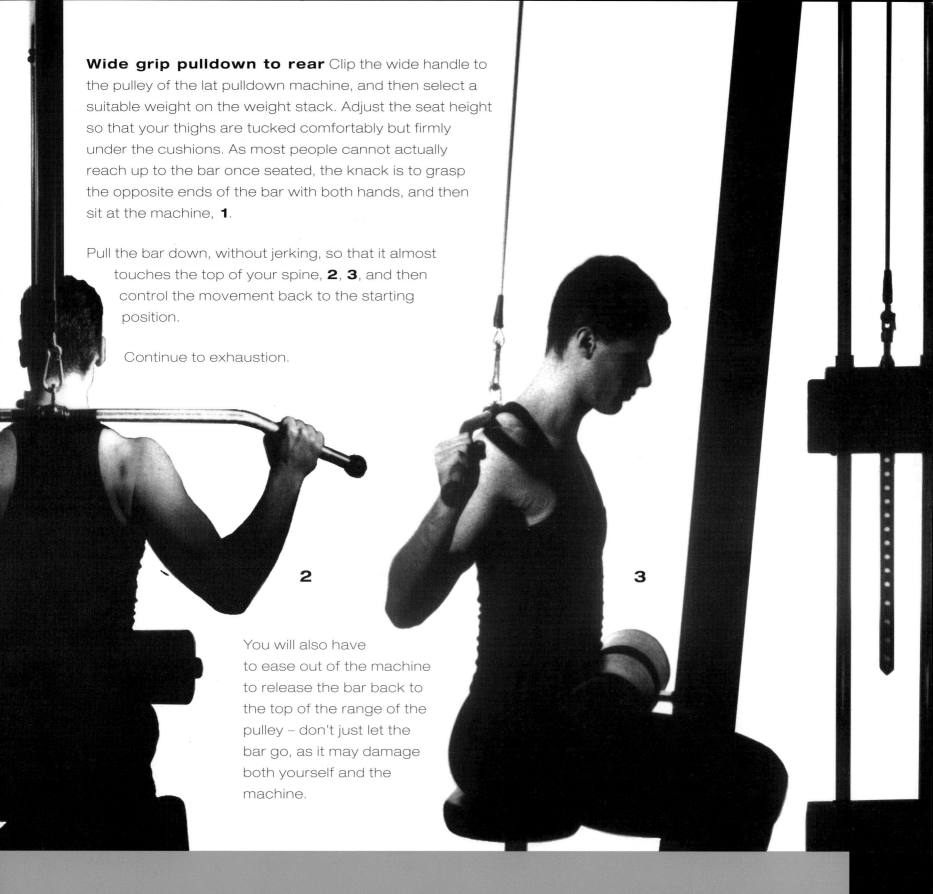

2

3

You will also have to ease out of the machine to release the bar back to the top of the range of the pulley – don't just let the bar go, as it may damage both yourself and the machine.

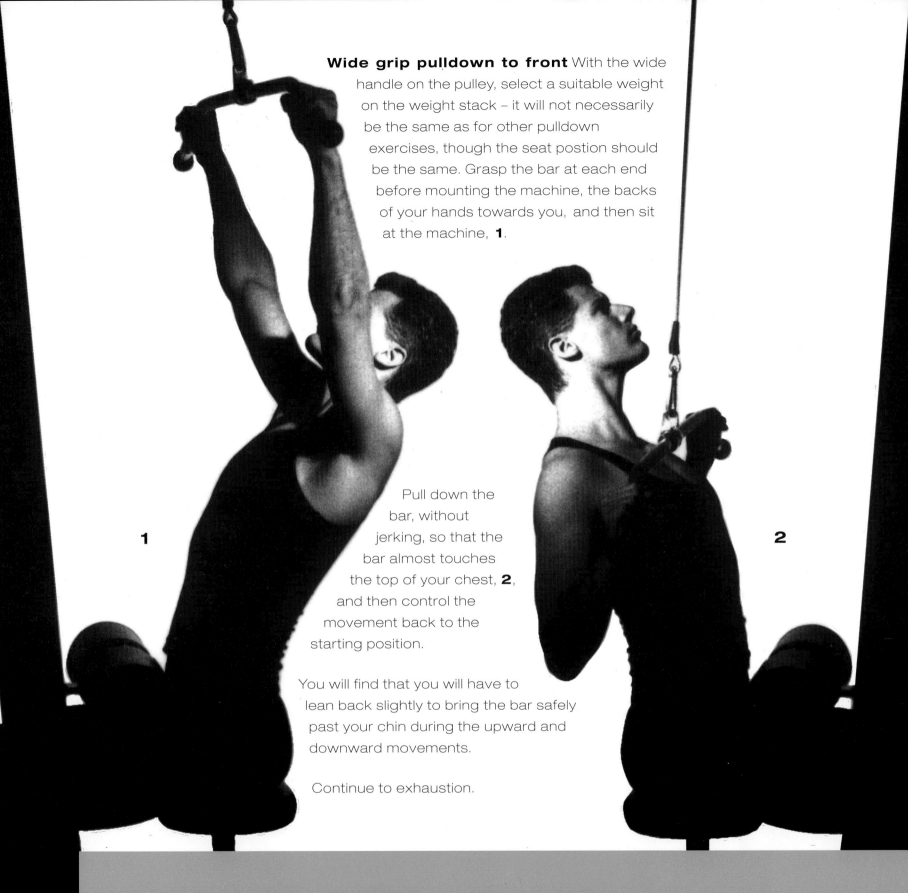

Wide grip pulldown to front With the wide handle on the pulley, select a suitable weight on the weight stack – it will not necessarily be the same as for other pulldown exercises, though the seat postion should be the same. Grasp the bar at each end before mounting the machine, the backs of your hands towards you, and then sit at the machine, **1**.

1

2

Pull down the bar, without jerking, so that the bar almost touches the top of your chest, **2**, and then control the movement back to the starting position.

You will find that you will have to lean back slightly to bring the bar safely past your chin during the upward and downward movements.

Continue to exhaustion.

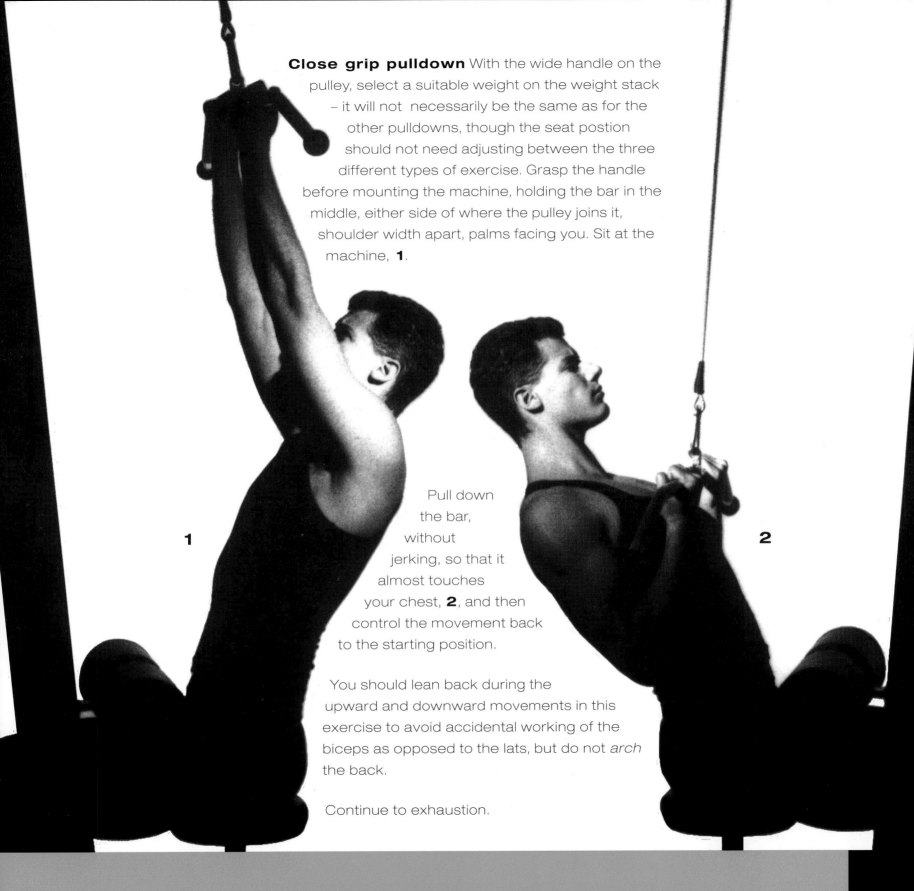

Close grip pulldown With the wide handle on the pulley, select a suitable weight on the weight stack – it will not necessarily be the same as for the other pulldowns, though the seat postion should not need adjusting between the three different types of exercise. Grasp the handle before mounting the machine, holding the bar in the middle, either side of where the pulley joins it, shoulder width apart, palms facing you. Sit at the machine, **1**.

1

2

Pull down the bar, without jerking, so that it almost touches your chest, **2**, and then control the movement back to the starting position.

You should lean back during the upward and downward movements in this exercise to avoid accidental working of the biceps as opposed to the lats, but do not *arch* the back.

Continue to exhaustion.

Pull-up In your gym you may find that for these exercises there is either a free-standing frame like the one shown here, or a wall-mounted version, which will probably have some steps or a mounting aid beneath. There are two versions of the pull-up. Both should be done to exhaustion, which will not take long.

Close grip pull-up Grasp the bar with palms facing you, the width of your face apart, and raise your body so that your chin just rises over the bar if you can, **1**.

Wide grip pull-up Grasp the bar with palms away from you, at the two ends of the bar, and then raise your body so that your chin again rises just above the bar, **2**.

Most people find these exercises extremely difficult, so many gyms have now installed an assisted pull-up machine, **3**, which effectively reduces you body weight to make the pull-up easier. Remember; the **more** weight you select the easier the exercise will be.

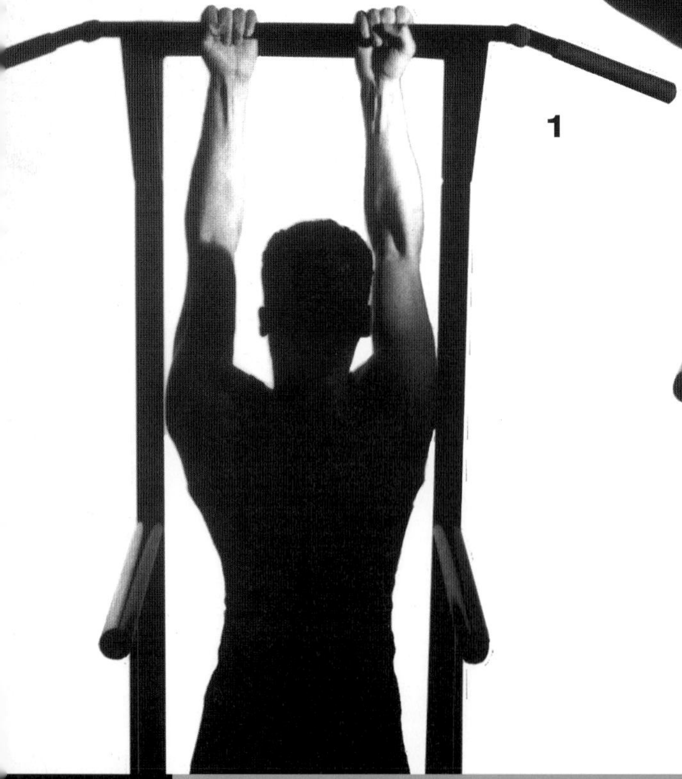

1

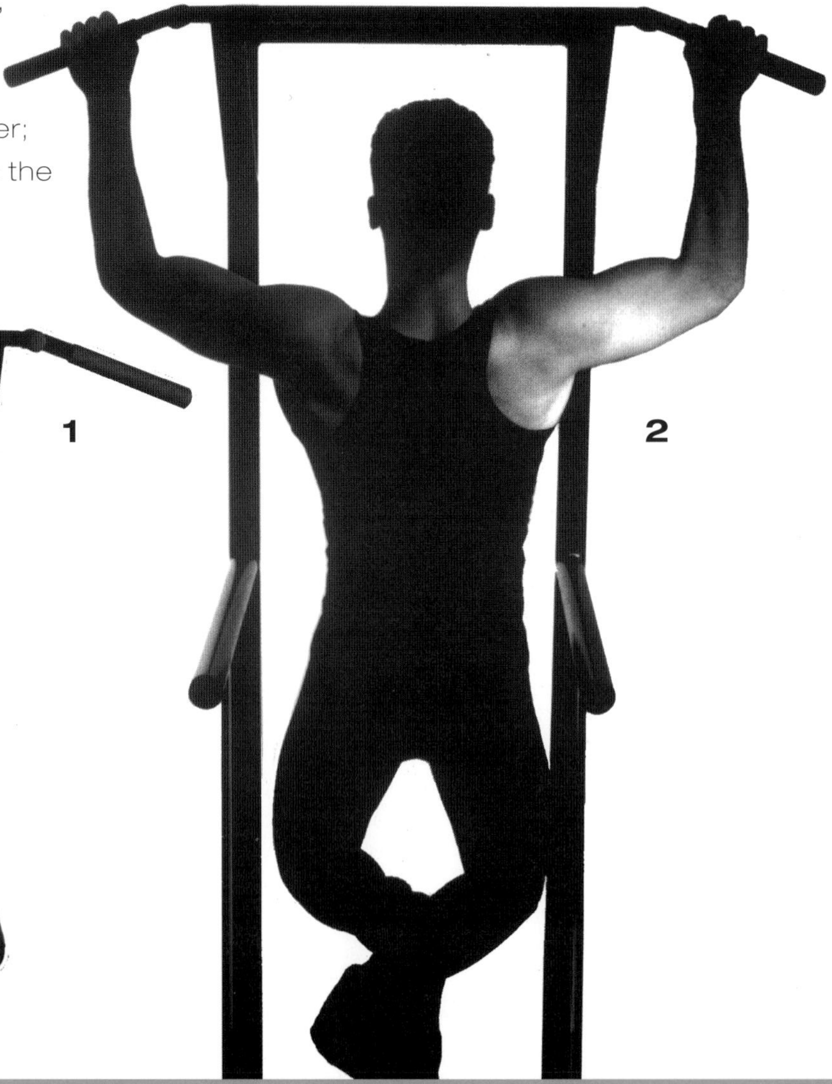

2

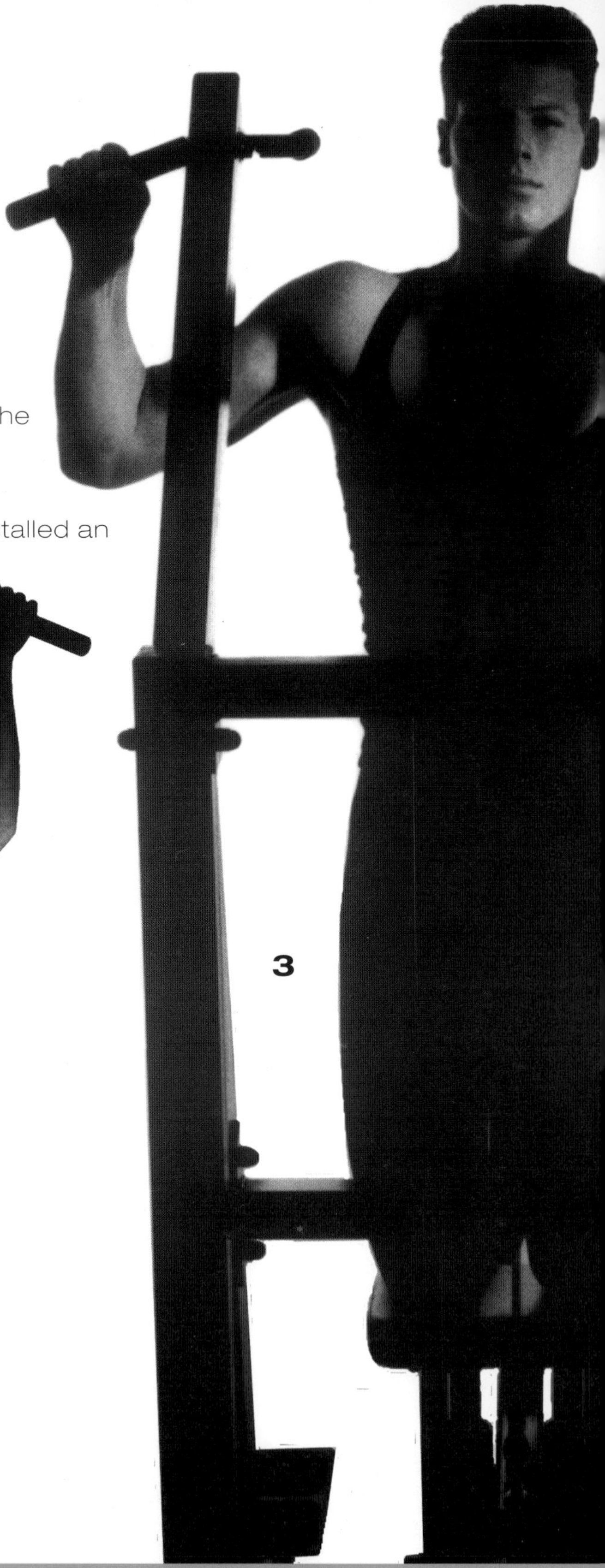

3

Bent-over row Select a suitable fixed barbell. Place on the floor in front of you, and then stand over it, knees bent, feet hip distance apart. Lean over and grasp the barbell slightly wider than shoulder distance apart with your hands, palms toward the bar, **1**.

Raise the bar towards your chest, **2**, with elbows out, and then control the downward movement to the starting position. **Your back should remain straight throughout.** Do not jerk the barbell upwards as you get towards exhaustion.

Try to keep the rest of the body stable during this exercise, which is actually very difficult to do. Performing this exercise in front of a mirror may help you to achieve this.

Continue to exhaustion.

Tightening your abdominals wil greatly help in keeping the lower back flat.

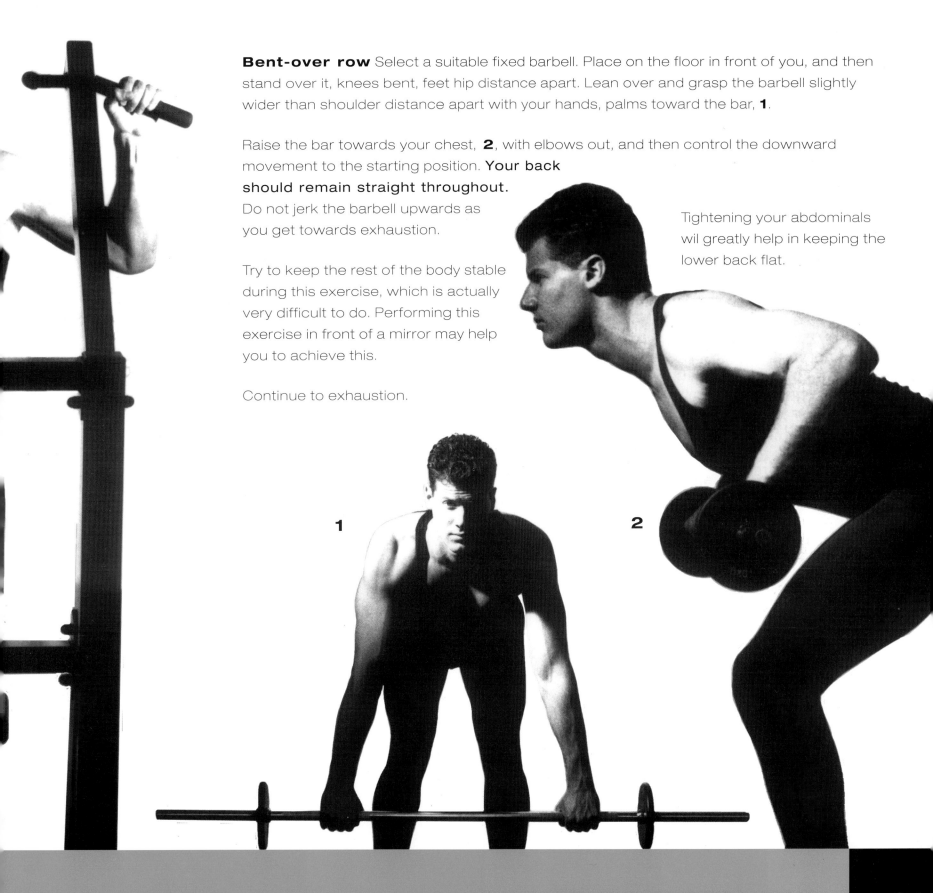

1

2

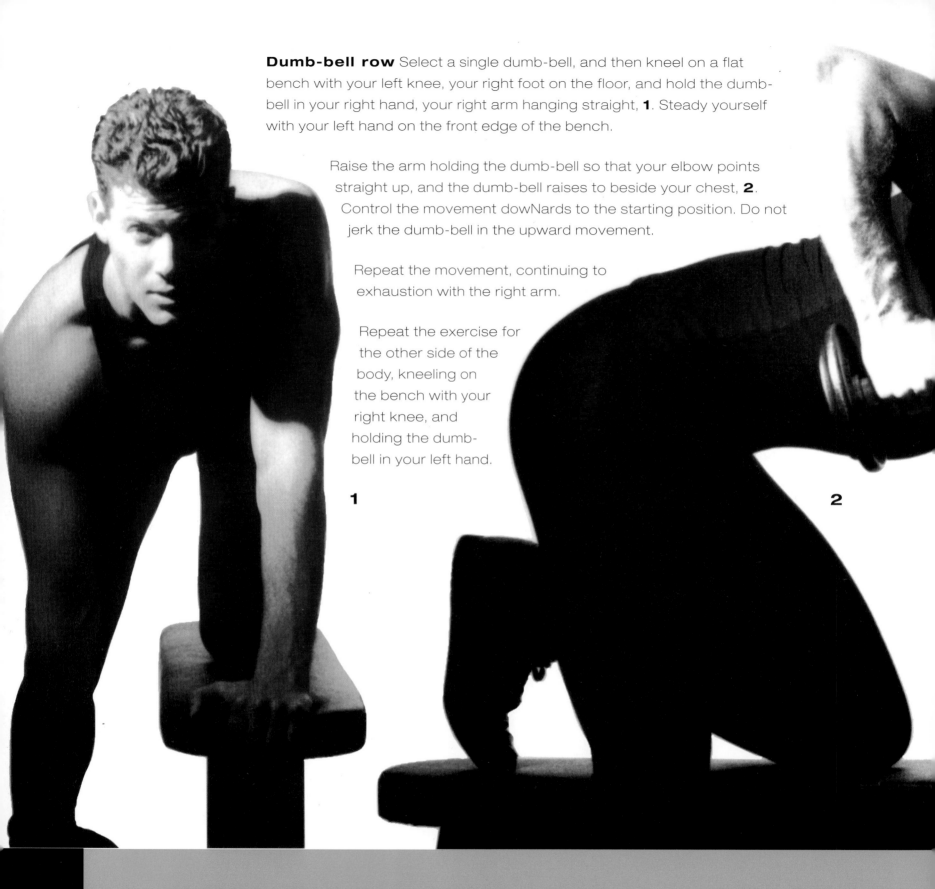

Dumb-bell row Select a single dumb-bell, and then kneel on a flat bench with your left knee, your right foot on the floor, and hold the dumb-bell in your right hand, your right arm hanging straight, **1**. Steady yourself with your left hand on the front edge of the bench.

Raise the arm holding the dumb-bell so that your elbow points straight up, and the dumb-bell raises to beside your chest, **2**. Control the movement dowNards to the starting position. Do not jerk the dumb-bell in the upward movement.

Repeat the movement, continuing to exhaustion with the right arm.

Repeat the exercise for the other side of the body, kneeling on the bench with your right knee, and holding the dumb-bell in your left hand.

1

2

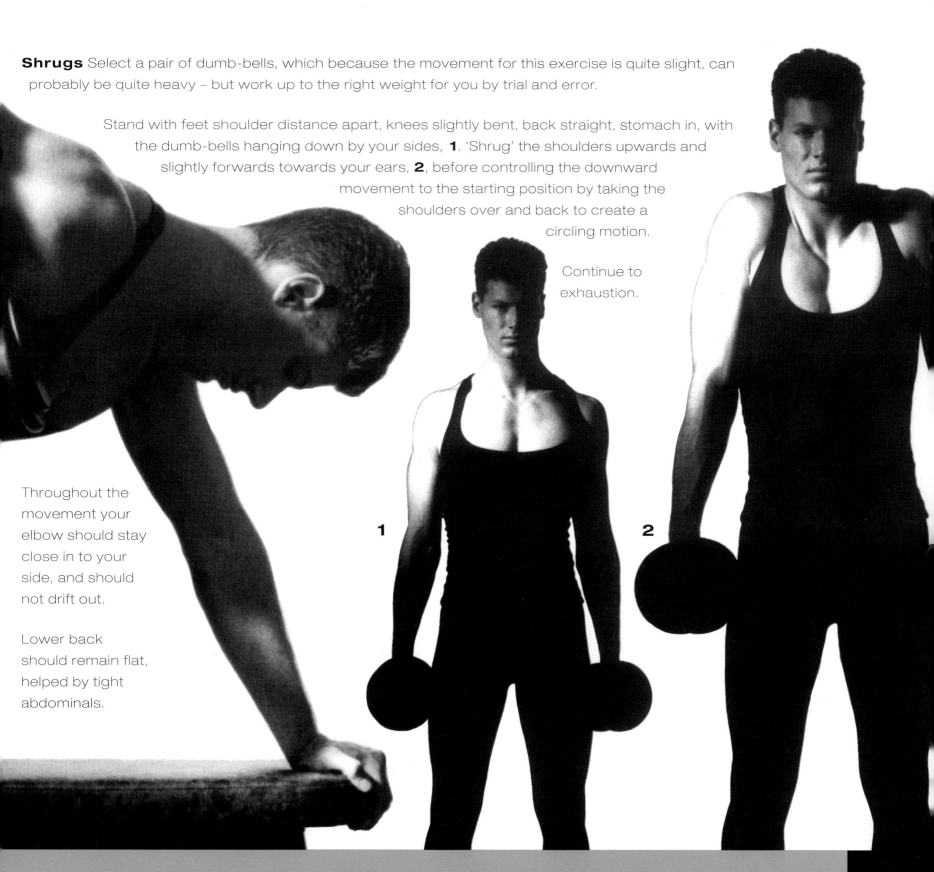

Shrugs Select a pair of dumb-bells, which because the movement for this exercise is quite slight, can probably be quite heavy – but work up to the right weight for you by trial and error.

Stand with feet shoulder distance apart, knees slightly bent, back straight, stomach in, with the dumb-bells hanging down by your sides, **1**. 'Shrug' the shoulders upwards and slightly forwards towards your ears, **2**, before controlling the downward movement to the starting position by taking the shoulders over and back to create a circling motion.

Continue to exhaustion.

Throughout the movement your elbow should stay close in to your side, and should not drift out.

Lower back should remain flat, helped by tight abdominals.

DUMB-BELL ROW/SHRUGS

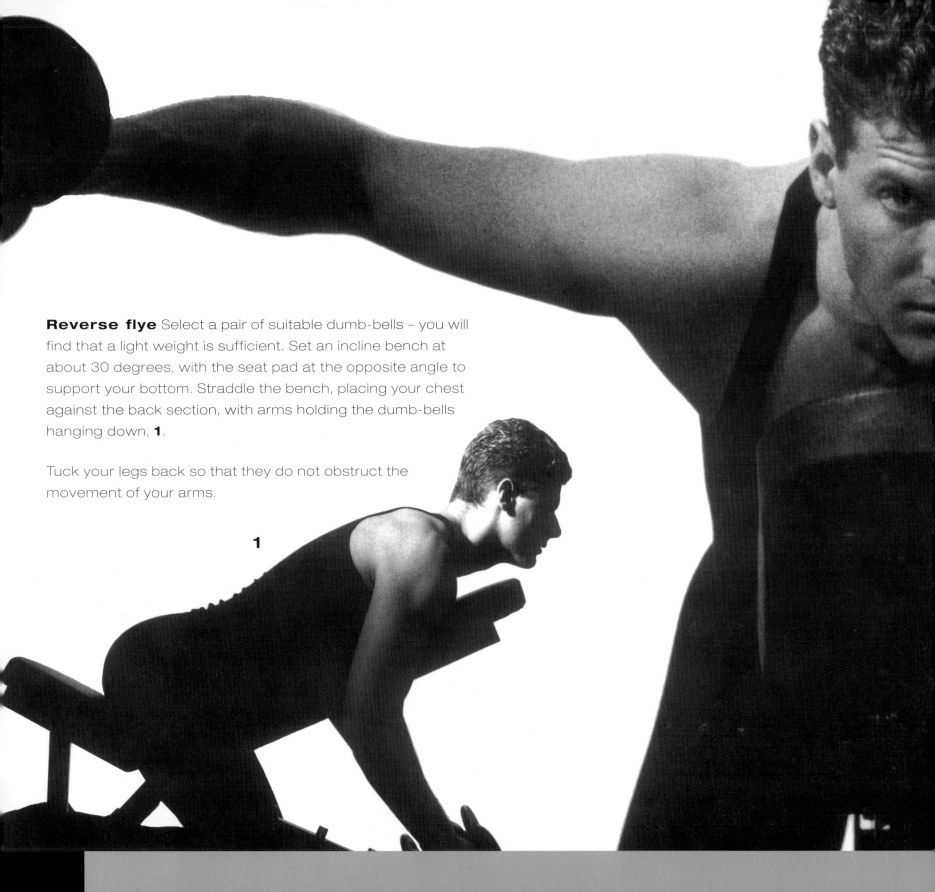

Reverse flye Select a pair of suitable dumb-bells – you will find that a light weight is sufficient. Set an incline bench at about 30 degrees, with the seat pad at the opposite angle to support your bottom. Straddle the bench, placing your chest against the back section, with arms holding the dumb-bells hanging down, **1**.

Tuck your legs back so that they do not obstruct the movement of your arms.

1

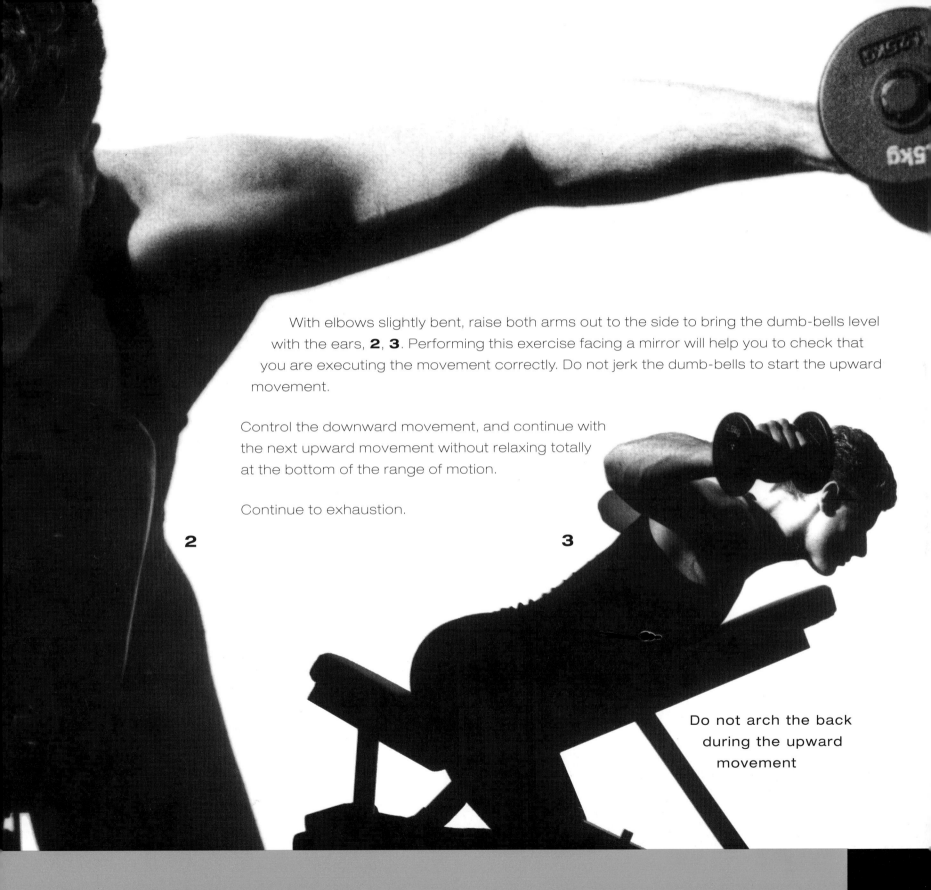

With elbows slightly bent, raise both arms out to the side to bring the dumb-bells level with the ears, **2**, **3**. Performing this exercise facing a mirror will help you to check that you are executing the movement correctly. Do not jerk the dumb-bells to start the upward movement.

Control the downward movement, and continue with the next upward movement without relaxing totally at the bottom of the range of motion.

Continue to exhaustion.

2

3

Do not arch the back during the upward movement

REVERSE FLYE

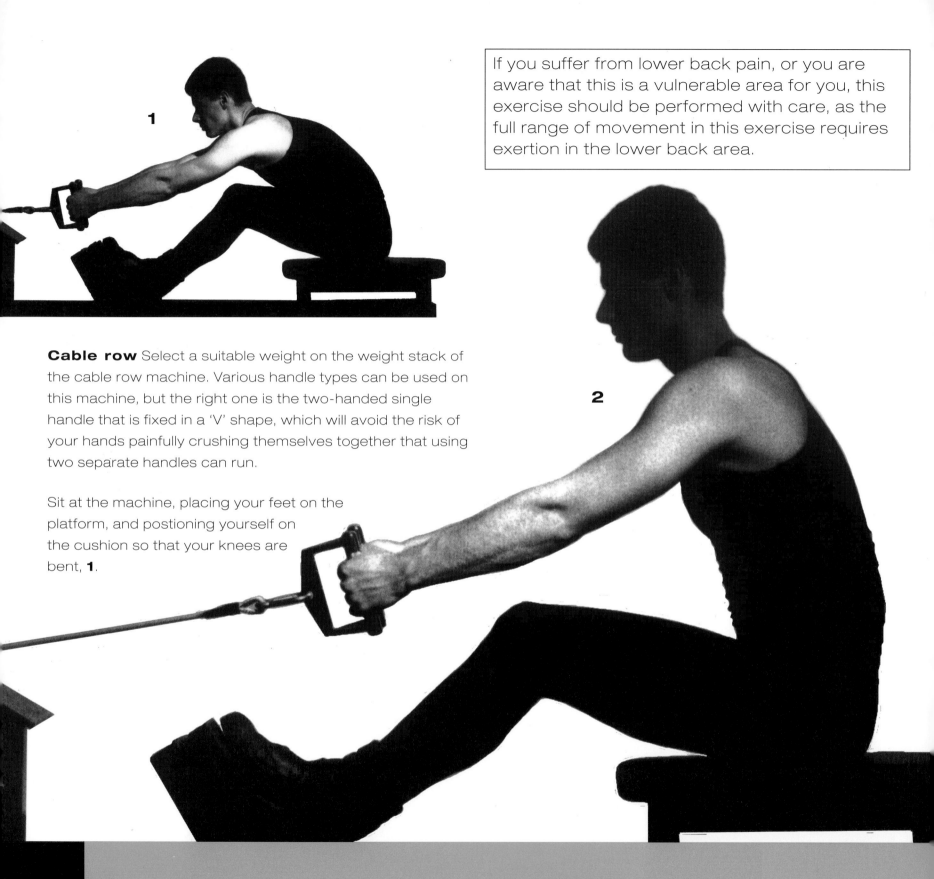

1

If you suffer from lower back pain, or you are aware that this is a vulnerable area for you, this exercise should be performed with care, as the full range of movement in this exercise requires exertion in the lower back area.

2

Cable row Select a suitable weight on the weight stack of the cable row machine. Various handle types can be used on this machine, but the right one is the two-handed single handle that is fixed in a 'V' shape, which will avoid the risk of your hands painfully crushing themselves together that using two separate handles can run.

Sit at the machine, placing your feet on the platform, and postioning yourself on the cushion so that your knees are bent, **1**.

Therefore, extreme care should be exercised by lower back injury sufferers to get to the upright position initially, and to release the cable again at the end of the exercise. For this reason, **only a light weight** should be selected on the weight stack, and the repetitions performed only as in **A** below.

Sit up from the starting position, at the same time drawing the arms up towards the body, **2**, continuing smoothly through to the final position where your hands are drawn to your stomach, and your back is straight and upright, **3**.

At this point you have two choices for the repetitions of this exercise:

A Keep back straight and upright, and control the movement of arms and shoulders only back and forth, or

B Return to position **2** (that is to say almost back to the starting position) working first your lower back, followed by your upper as you complete the movement to postition **3**.

Whichever you choose (note that it is B which is dangerous for lower back pain sufferers) continue to exhaustion, returning the handle to the release point with care.

Remember to keep your abdominals in tight, and your elbows by your sides, and that you must not not lean back.

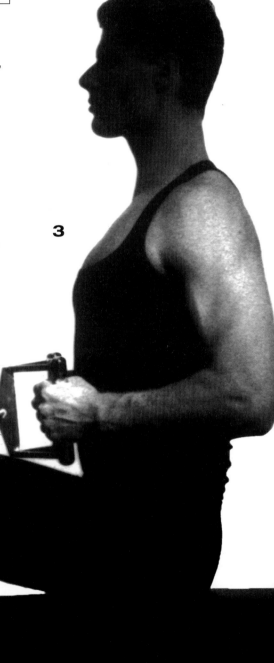

3

Back extension To perform this exercise safely and well you must use a piece of equipment known as a Roman chair. There are two types, upright and inclined. The safest and best is the incline type, as the resistance to gravity (which is effectively what the exercise involves) is slightly less than for the upright Roman chair, and lower back injury through over-stress is what you want to avoid.

Adjust the cushion height of the chair so that it is comfortably against the upper thighs and lower stomach area, but not so high that the bend forward will be difficult. Mount the machine, and after first using your hands to support your upper body as you get your balance, raise them to place your knuckles lightly against your temples, **1**.

Bend forward, keeping your back straight at all times, until your legs and back form a right angle, **2**. Do **not over-extend to lower than this.**

Return to the starting position, then continue the movement to exhaustion.

If you suffer from lower back pain do not perform this exercise.

You may see others performing this exercise with a weight held behind the neck to increase the workload. **This is not recommended.**

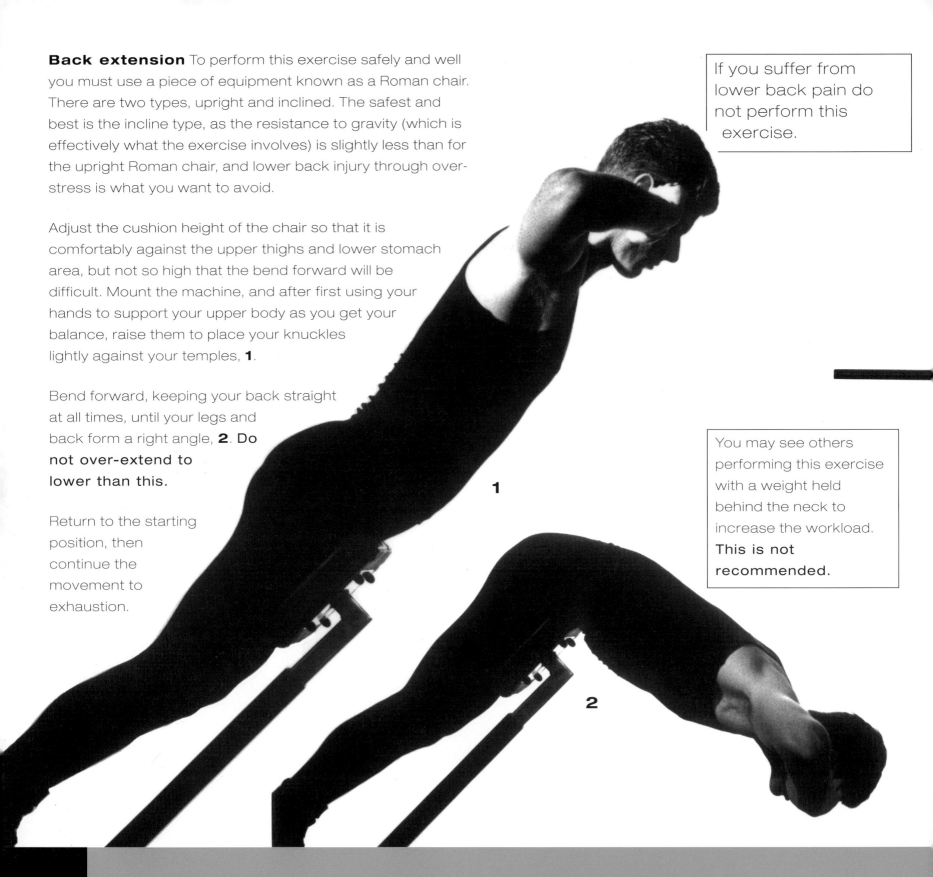

'Good morning' This exercise is performed with a fixed barbell, which does not need to be heavy to produce an effective result.

Stand with feet wider than shoulder distance apart, knees slightly bent, back straight, stomach in, having first hoisted the barbell across your shoulders, partly supporting its weight with your arms to avoid discomfort at the back of your neck, **1**.

Bend forward, all the while keeping your back straight, **2**, continuing on past this point if you feel comfortable, until your upper body is parallel to the floor, **3**.

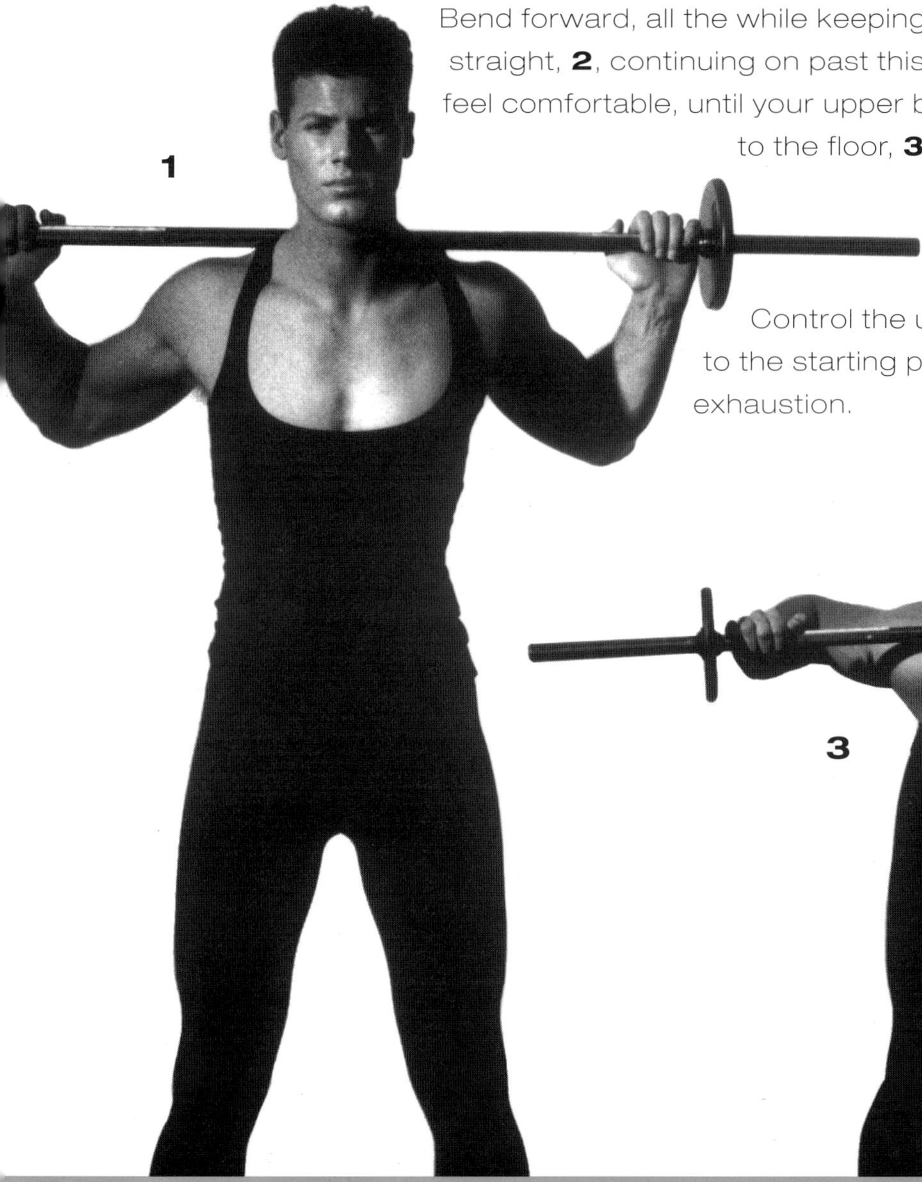

Control the upward movement back to the starting position, and then continue to exhaustion.

If you suffer from lower back pain do not perform this exercise.

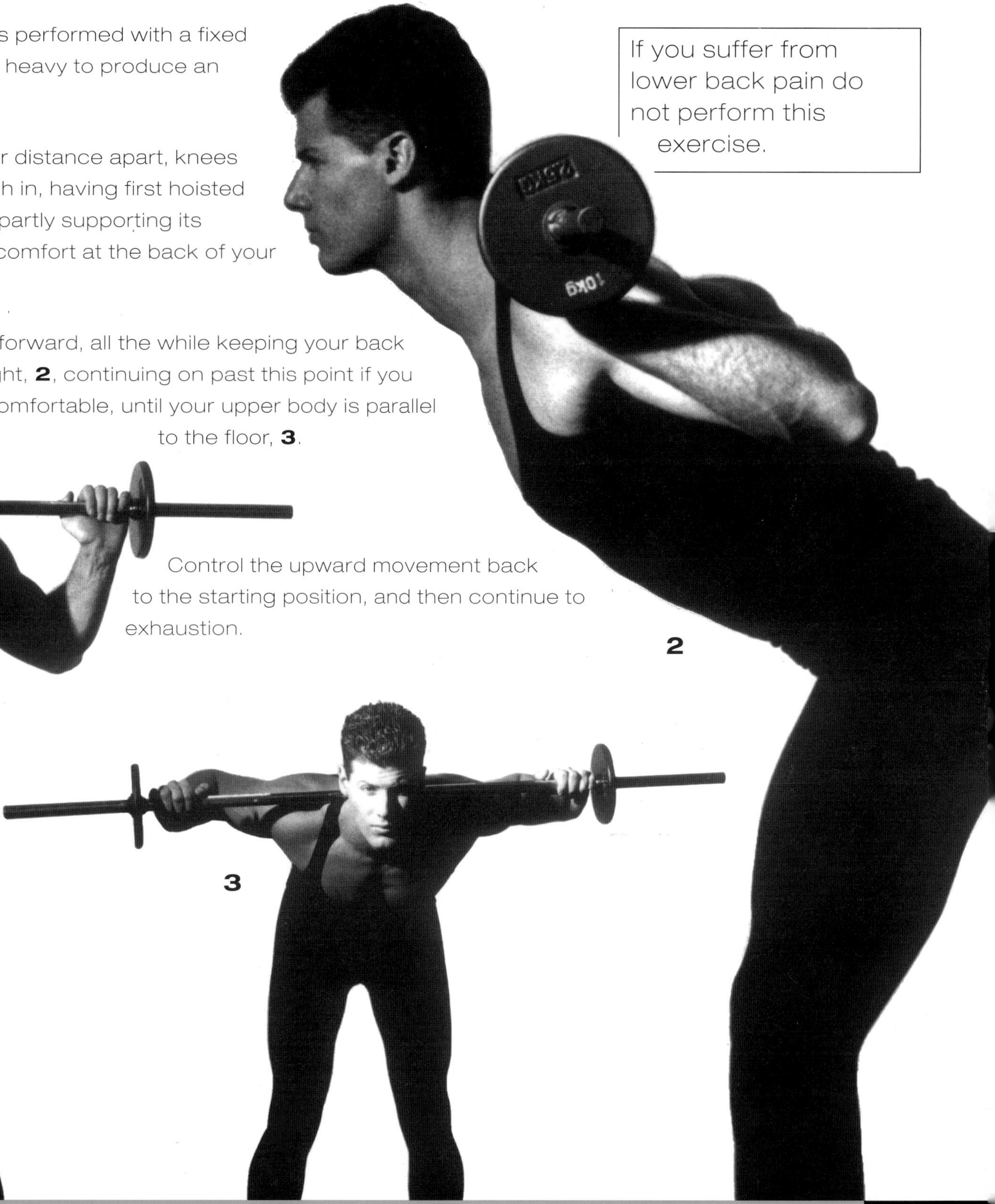

1

2

3

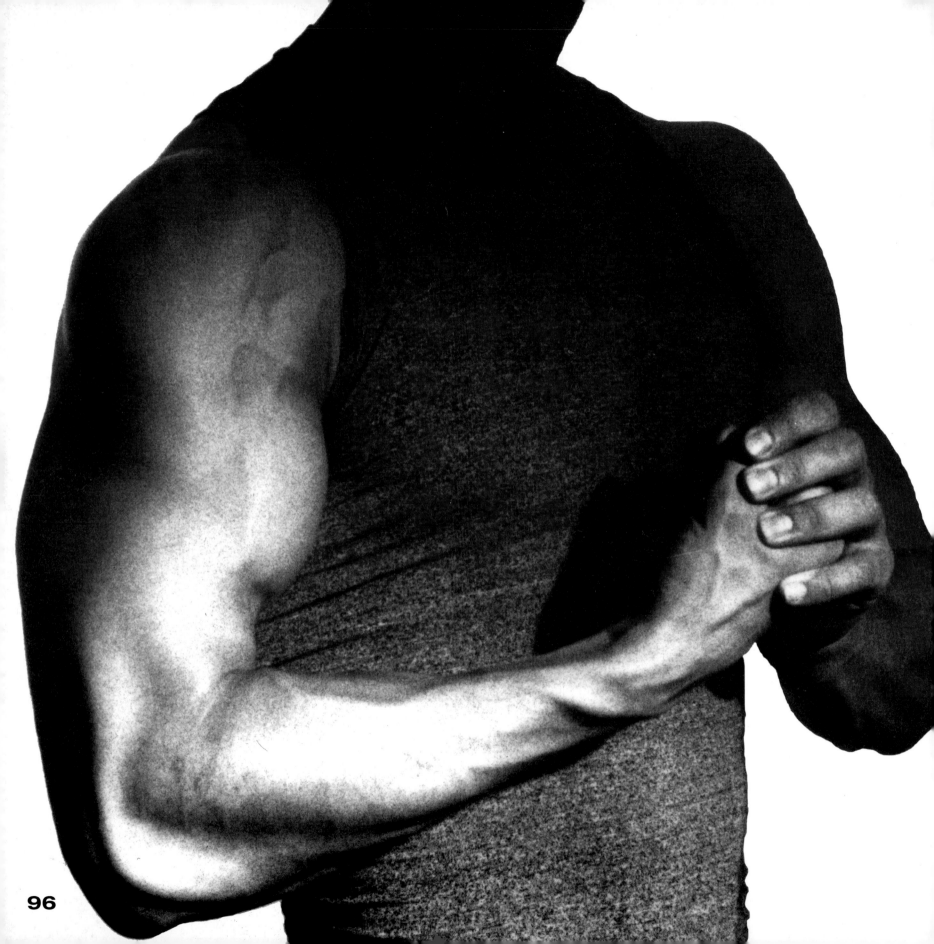

The group of muscles in the arms are arguably the most frequently displayed, and so the wise owner makes keeping these prominent assets in good order a high priority.

SERVICING OF MOVING PARTS **ARMS**

The two key muscles are the **bicep** (the bulging curved one on the front of the upper arm) and the **tricep** (the forked one on the back of the upper arm).

Section essentials

All exercises should be performed to exhaustion, i.e. to the point at which you cannot achieve another rep.

The weight selected should be chosen to achieve the following ratio of reps and sets for *either*

Endurance work:
2–3 sets of 15–20 reps

or

Muscle building work:
3–5 sets of 6–8 reps

Rest between sets for only the length of time it has taken you to perform the previous set.

Take a deep breath prior to starting an exercise, then exhale on the <u>exertion</u> and inhale on the <u>recovery</u>. Do not hold your breath – this may dangerously elevate the blood pressure.

Where your arms are working towards being straight, take care not to '<u>lock out</u>'. Keep limbs slightly bent.

Explore possibilities beyond the exercises shown. Ask for instruction on <u>isolation machines</u> available for specific body parts that you can add into your programme for variety.

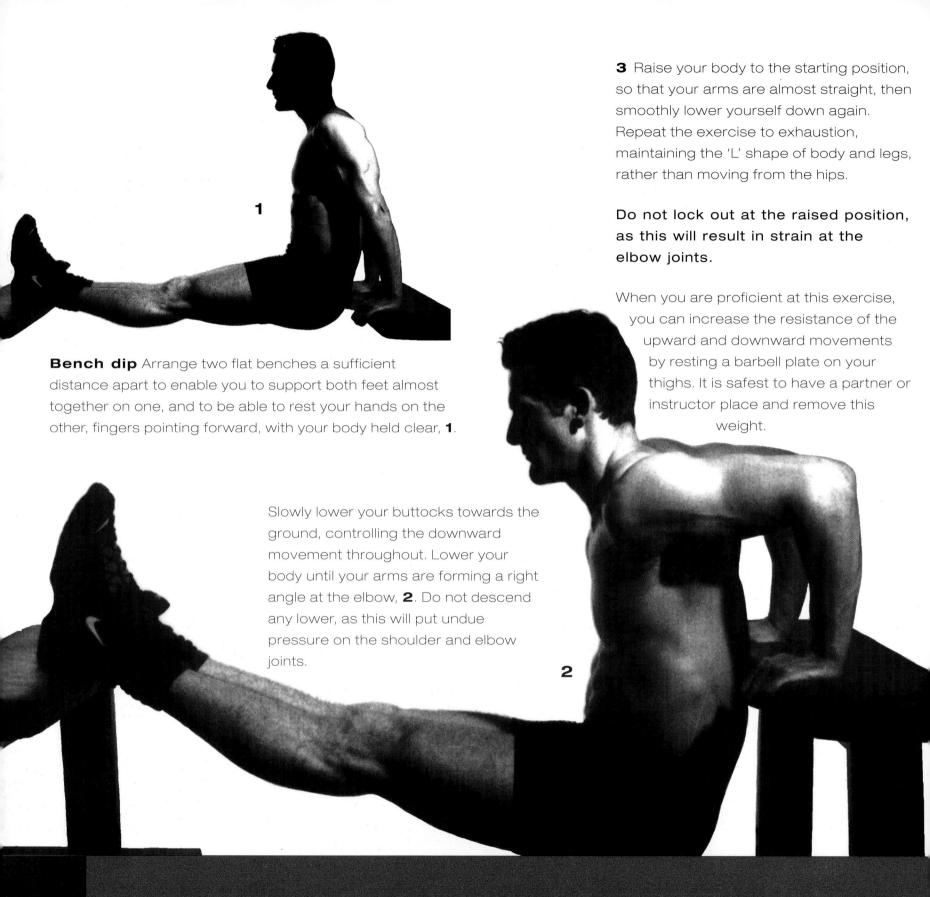

3 Raise your body to the starting position, so that your arms are almost straight, then smoothly lower yourself down again. Repeat the exercise to exhaustion, maintaining the 'L' shape of body and legs, rather than moving from the hips.

Do not lock out at the raised position, as this will result in strain at the elbow joints.

When you are proficient at this exercise, you can increase the resistance of the upward and downward movements by resting a barbell plate on your thighs. It is safest to have a partner or instructor place and remove this weight.

Bench dip Arrange two flat benches a sufficient distance apart to enable you to support both feet almost together on one, and to be able to rest your hands on the other, fingers pointing forward, with your body held clear, **1**.

Slowly lower your buttocks towards the ground, controlling the downward movement throughout. Lower your body until your arms are forming a right angle at the elbow, **2**. Do not descend any lower, as this will put undue pressure on the shoulder and elbow joints.

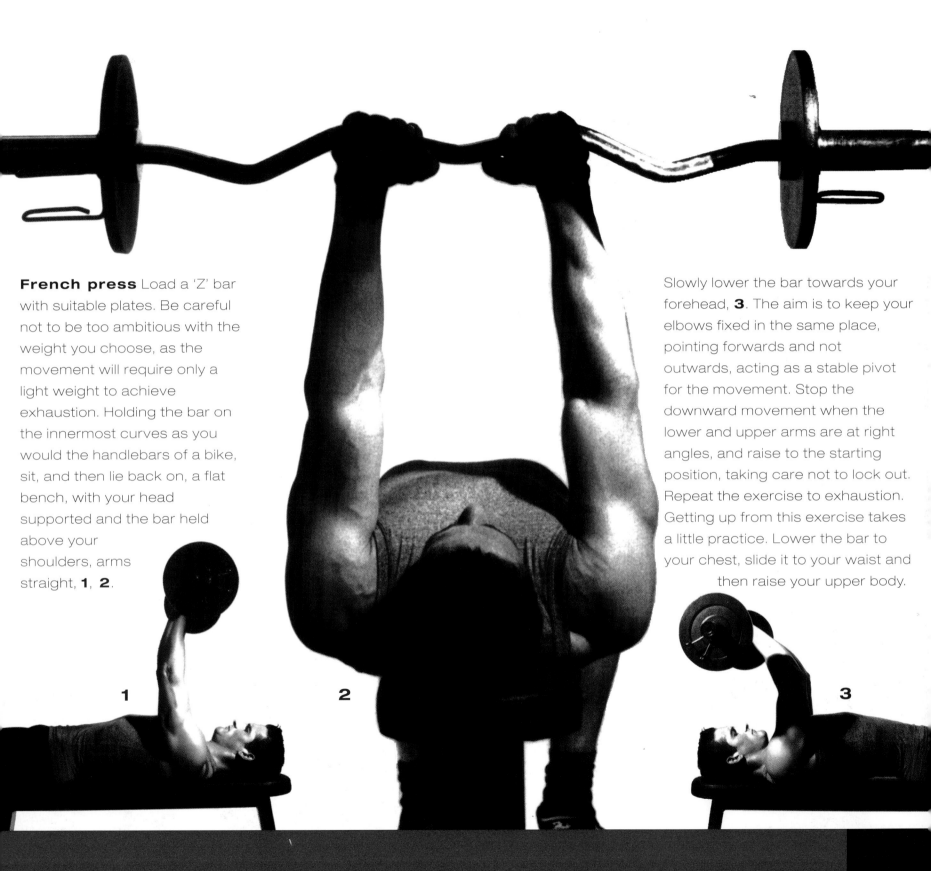

French press Load a 'Z' bar with suitable plates. Be careful not to be too ambitious with the weight you choose, as the movement will require only a light weight to achieve exhaustion. Holding the bar on the innermost curves as you would the handlebars of a bike, sit, and then lie back on, a flat bench, with your head supported and the bar held above your shoulders, arms straight, **1**, **2**.

Slowly lower the bar towards your forehead, **3**. The aim is to keep your elbows fixed in the same place, pointing forwards and not outwards, acting as a stable pivot for the movement. Stop the downward movement when the lower and upper arms are at right angles, and raise to the starting position, taking care not to lock out. Repeat the exercise to exhaustion. Getting up from this exercise takes a little practice. Lower the bar to your chest, slide it to your waist and then raise your upper body.

1

2

3

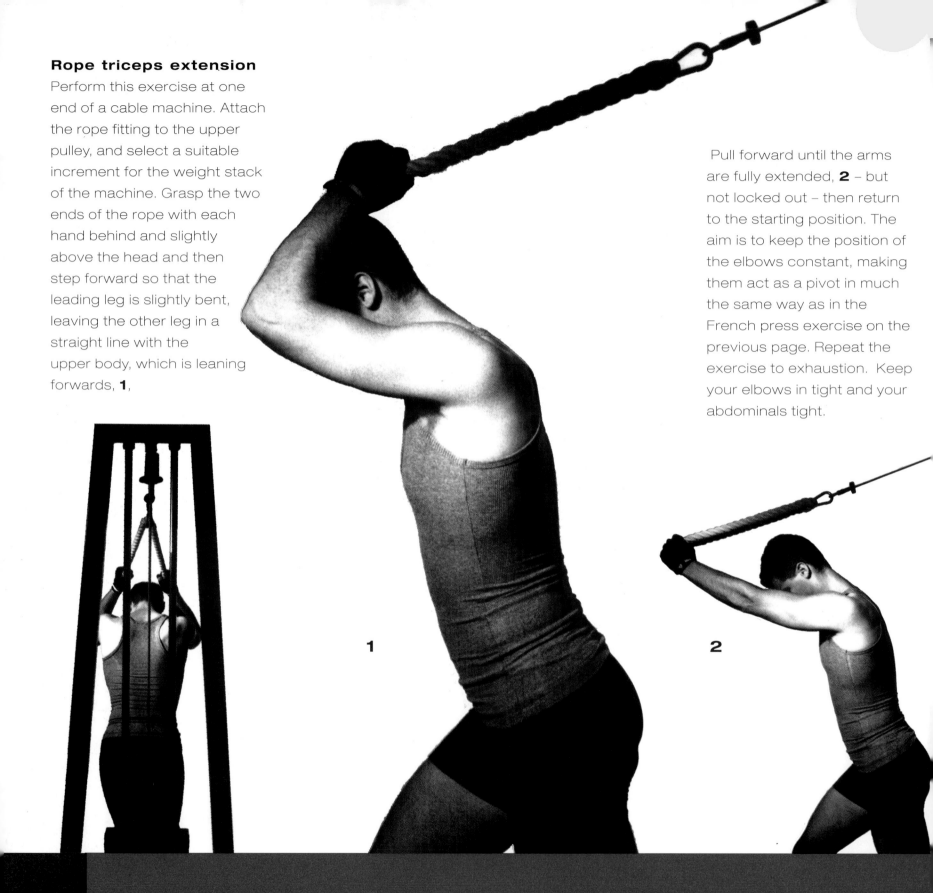

Rope triceps extension

Perform this exercise at one end of a cable machine. Attach the rope fitting to the upper pulley, and select a suitable increment for the weight stack of the machine. Grasp the two ends of the rope with each hand behind and slightly above the head and then step forward so that the leading leg is slightly bent, leaving the other leg in a straight line with the upper body, which is leaning forwards, **1**,

Pull forward until the arms are fully extended, **2** – but not locked out – then return to the starting position. The aim is to keep the position of the elbows constant, making them act as a pivot in much the same way as in the French press exercise on the previous page. Repeat the exercise to exhaustion. Keep your elbows in tight and your abdominals tight.

1

2

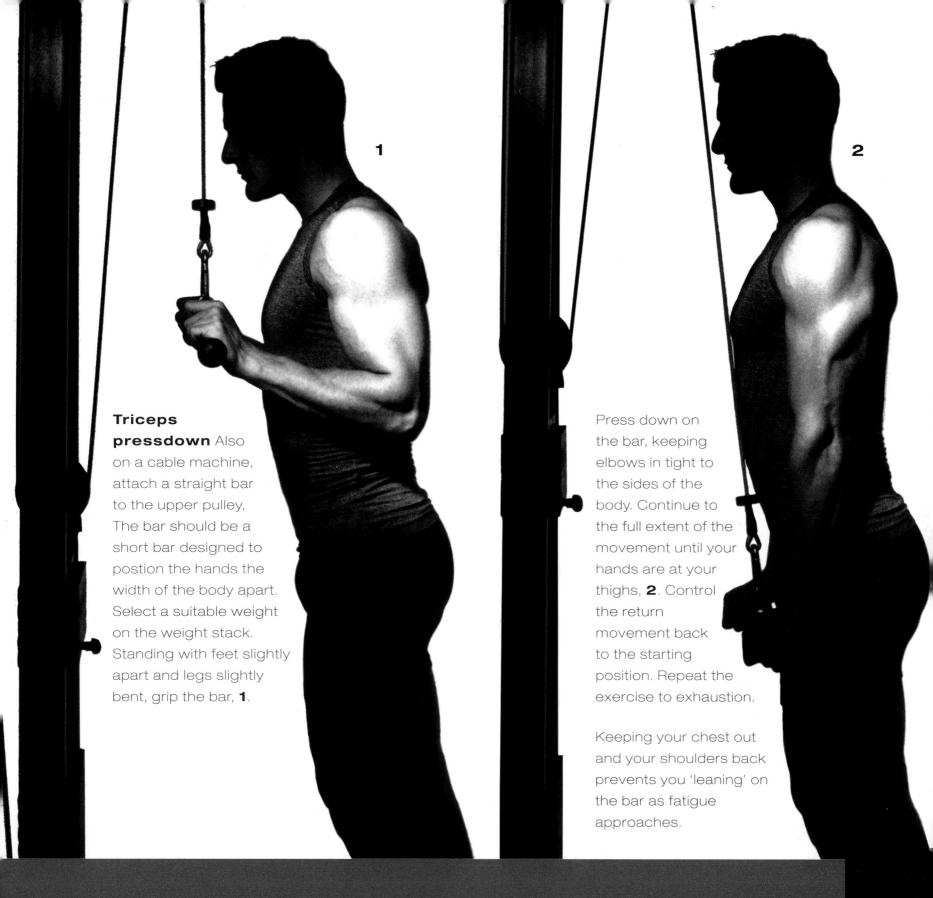

Triceps pressdown Also on a cable machine, attach a straight bar to the upper pulley, The bar should be a short bar designed to postion the hands the width of the body apart. Select a suitable weight on the weight stack. Standing with feet slightly apart and legs slightly bent, grip the bar, **1**.

Press down on the bar, keeping elbows in tight to the sides of the body. Continue to the full extent of the movement until your hands are at your thighs, **2**. Control the return movement back to the starting position. Repeat the exercise to exhaustion.

Keeping your chest out and your shoulders back prevents you 'leaning' on the bar as fatigue approaches.

Dumb-bell kick-back Select a suitable dumb-bell, after first getting a feel for the correct weight for you by starting with the lightest available.

Holding the dumb-bell in your right hand, position your left hand, left knee and left foot on a flat bench, with your right leg bent, your balance steadied with your right foot.

Your back should be straight, and your upper and lower arm at right angles to each other with the dumb-bell straight down, **1**.

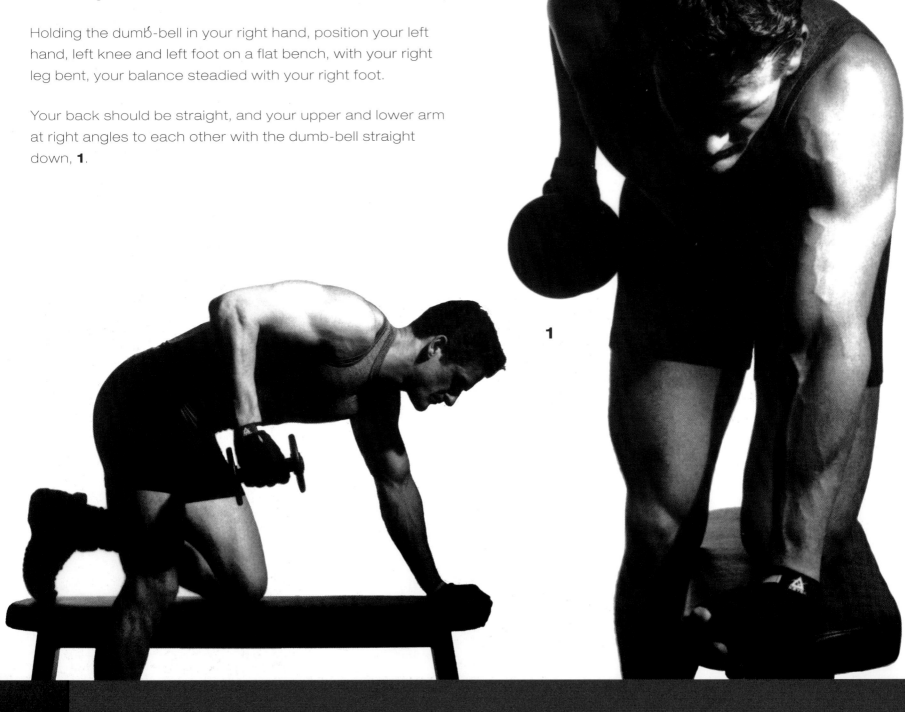

1

Keeping your upper arm steady, and your elbow fixed as the pivot, raise the dumb-bell backwards until your arm is straight, **2**. Lower the weight, controlling the return movement throughout. Repeat the exercise to exhaustion.

Do not swing the weight backwards, or lock out when your arm is straight. Repeat the exercise for the other arm, postioning the opposite knee, hand and foot on the other side of the bench.

You may find it useful to do this exercise side-on to a mirror so that for the first few times you can check that your upper arm and elbow are held steady.

As you approach fatigue, the tendency is to twist the upper body towards the dumb-bell side to give extra momentum. This is very dangerous, as the joints of the spine are 'open' in this flexed position.

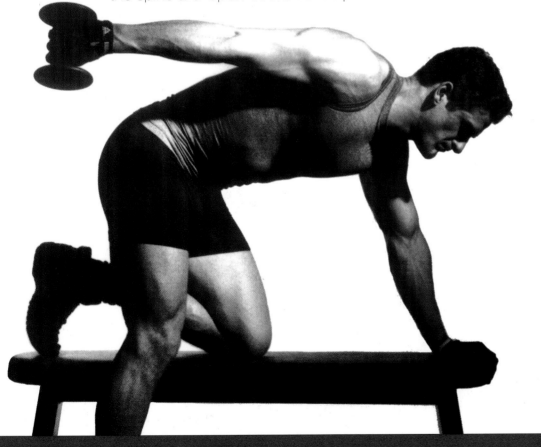

2

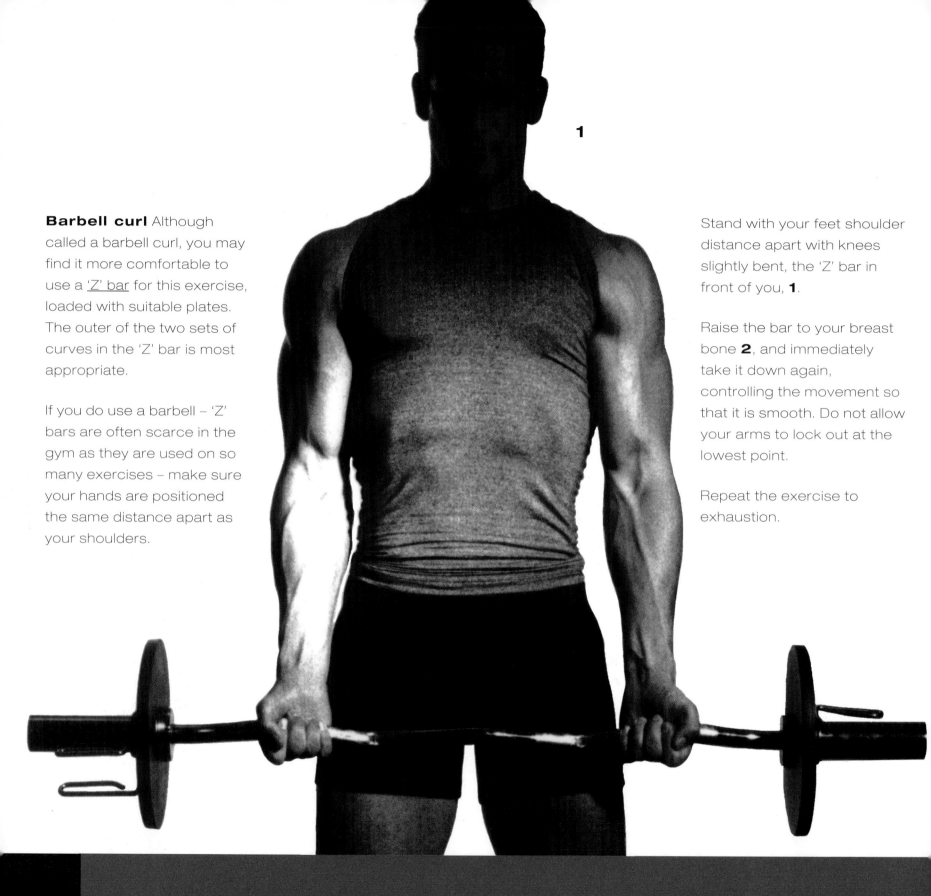

Barbell curl Although called a barbell curl, you may find it more comfortable to use a 'Z' bar for this exercise, loaded with suitable plates. The outer of the two sets of curves in the 'Z' bar is most appropriate.

If you do use a barbell – 'Z' bars are often scarce in the gym as they are used on so many exercises – make sure your hands are positioned the same distance apart as your shoulders.

Stand with your feet shoulder distance apart with knees slightly bent, the 'Z' bar in front of you, **1**.

Raise the bar to your breast bone **2**, and immediately take it down again, controlling the movement so that it is smooth. Do not allow your arms to lock out at the lowest point.

Repeat the exercise to exhaustion.

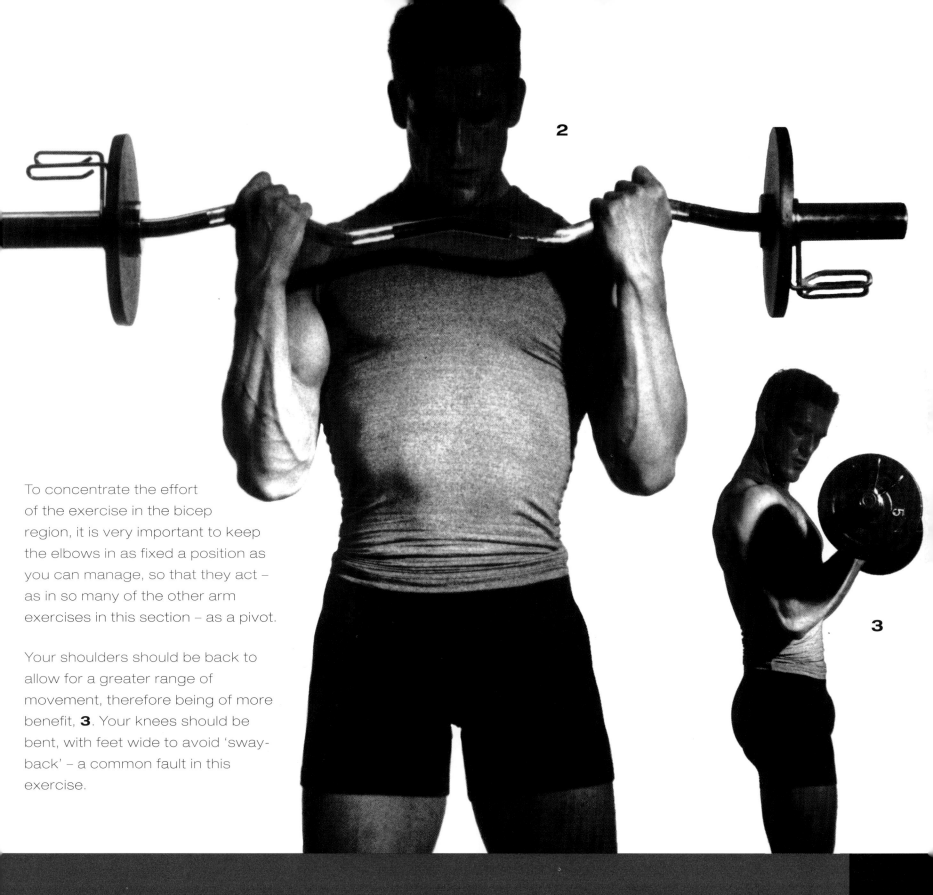

2

3

To concentrate the effort of the exercise in the bicep region, it is very important to keep the elbows in as fixed a position as you can manage, so that they act – as in so many of the other arm exercises in this section – as a pivot.

Your shoulders should be back to allow for a greater range of movement, therefore being of more benefit, **3**. Your knees should be bent, with feet wide to avoid 'sway-back' – a common fault in this exercise.

Close-grip preacher curl Select suitable plates for a 'Z' bar, and before starting the exercise, check that the seat at the <u>preacher bench</u> is adjusted to the right height. The crest of the arm pad should not be too tight under your armpits.

From the starting position, **1**, raise the bar until the lower arms are vertical, **2**.

Without losing motion, lower smoothly back to the starting postion, where you should not lock out.

Repeat the exercise to exhaustion.

Your elbows should stay in contact with the arm pad at all times, and you should avoid the tendency to lift your buttocks off the seat.

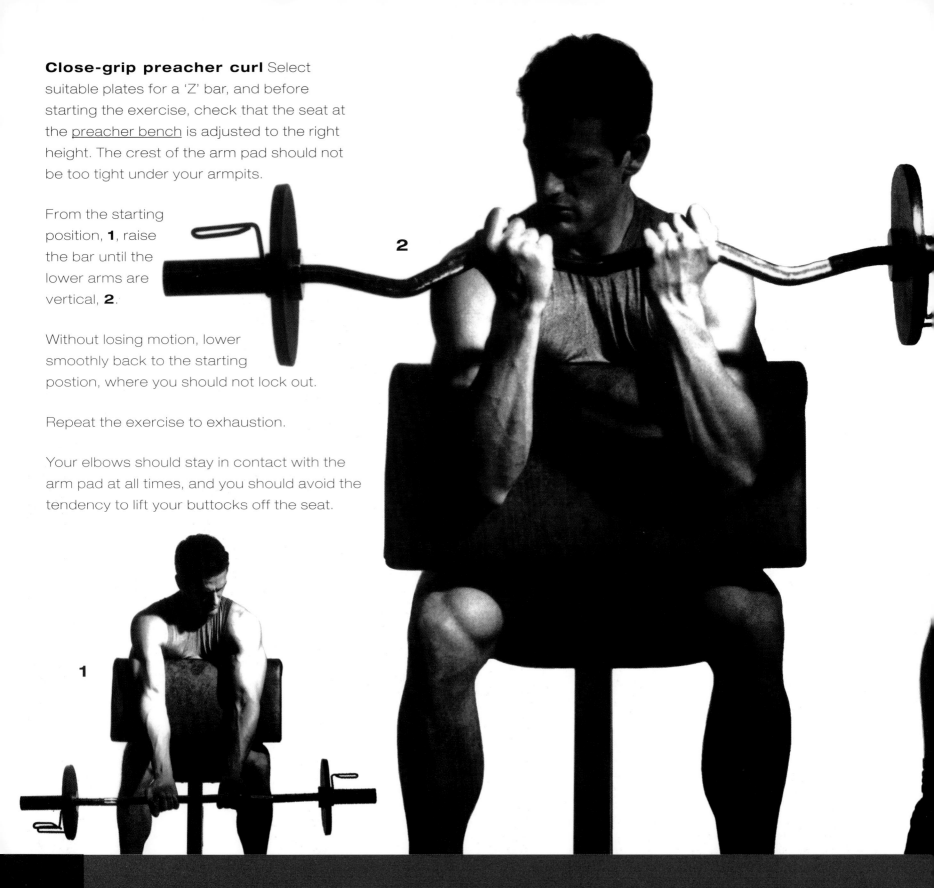

Dumb-bell concentration curl Sit on the end of a flat bench, with legs apart, and feet firmly placed, having selected a suitable dumb-bell. Grip the dumb-bell with your right hand and support the elbow against the inside of your right knee. Support your back with the non-working left arm, by placing your hand on your left knee, pressing down, **1**.

From the starting position, raise the dumb-bell up towards the opposite side of your chest, keeping the elbow fixed against the knee, **2**.

Lower the dumb-bell, controlling the downward movement. Do not lock out at the bottom.

Continue the exercise to exhaustion, then repeat with the left arm.

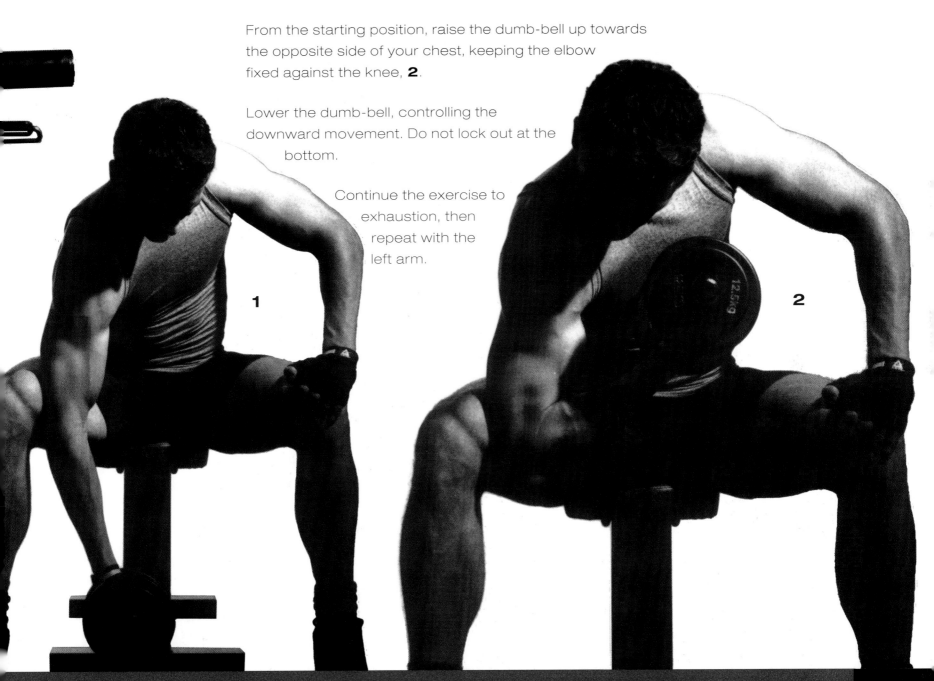

Seated alternate dumb-bell curl Select a pair of suitable dumb-bells, and then sit at either an up-righted incline bench, set so that the seat is parallel to the floor and the back is at right angles to it, or a bench specifically designed for this purpose. These are becoming increasingly available in gyms.

From the starting position, arms slightly bent, **1**, raise your right arm to your right shoulder, **2**, then control the lowering of the dumb-bell to the starting position, taking care not to lock out at the bottom.

You may turn the head to look at the bicep. This will allow you to check on the 'twist'.

Repeat the same motion with your left arm to your left shoulder, **3**.

The rhythm of the exercise should mean that you are starting the upward motion of one arm within a split second of the previous arm's downward movement being complete.

Continue the exercise to exhaustion.

Your palms should face in towards your body, and you should twist the hand as it comes up to shoulder height so that the little finger side comes toward your face. This 'twist' is vital since the bicep is responsible for this movement, as well as rasing the arm at the elbow.

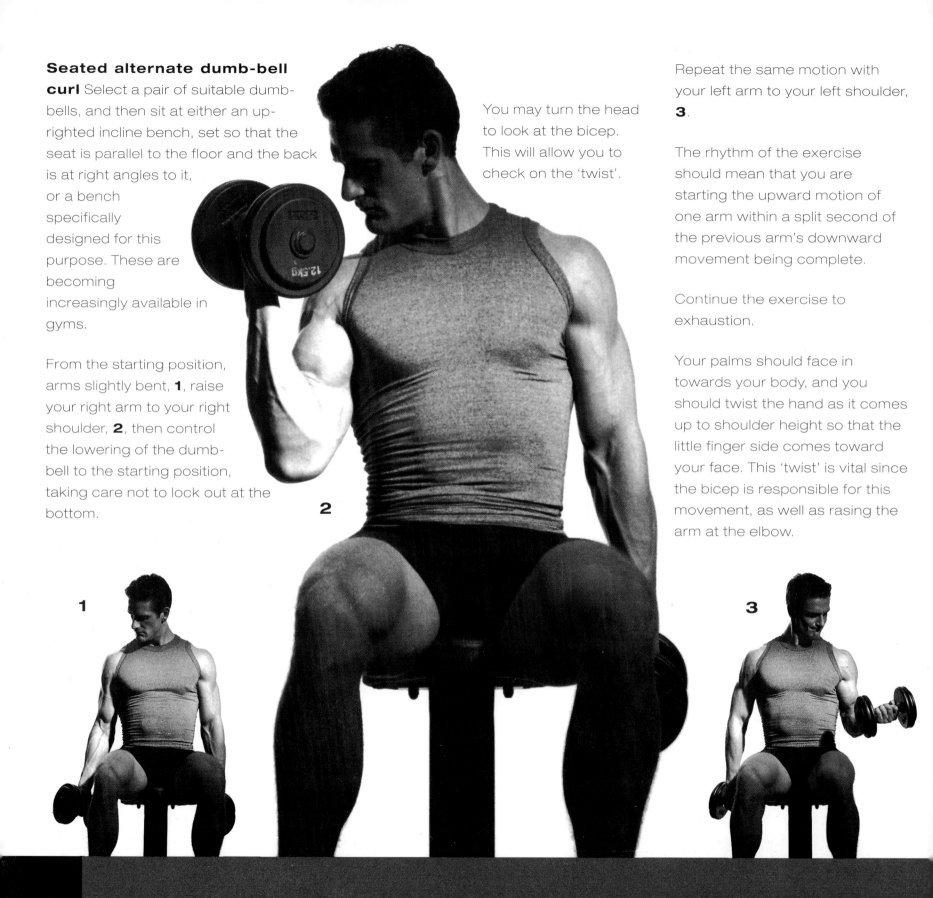

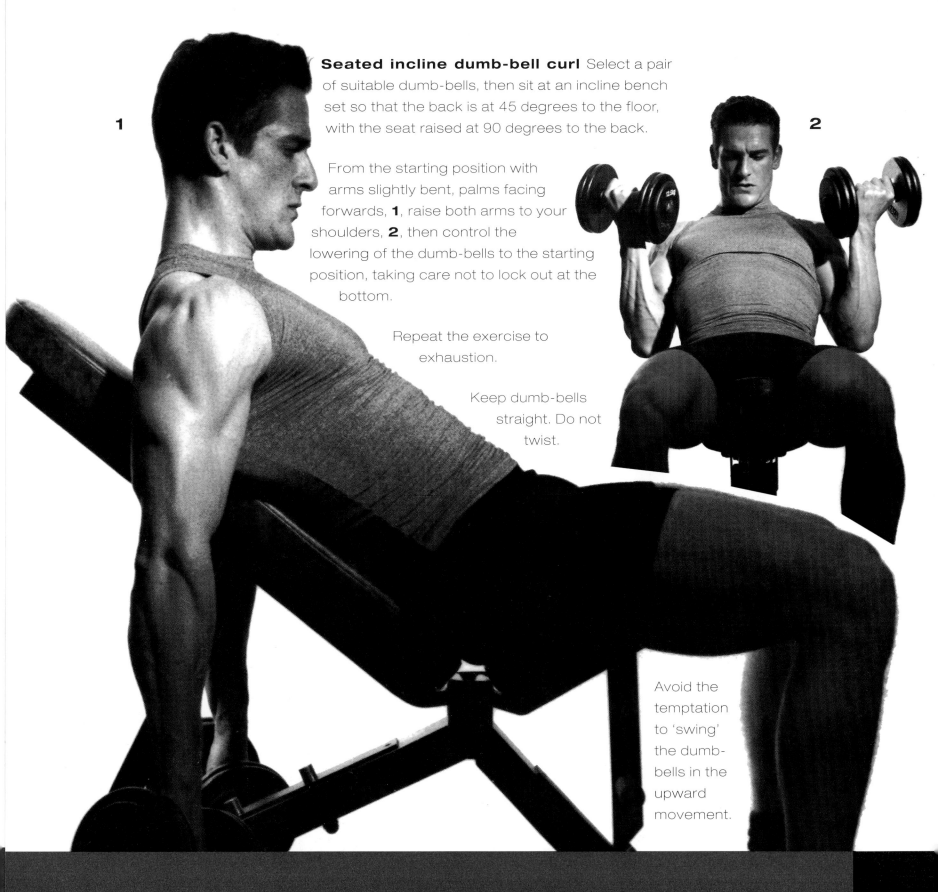

1

2

Seated incline dumb-bell curl Select a pair of suitable dumb-bells, then sit at an incline bench set so that the back is at 45 degrees to the floor, with the seat raised at 90 degrees to the back.

From the starting position with arms slightly bent, palms facing forwards, **1**, raise both arms to your shoulders, **2**, then control the lowering of the dumb-bells to the starting position, taking care not to lock out at the bottom.

Repeat the exercise to exhaustion.

Keep dumb-bells straight. Do not twist.

Avoid the temptation to 'swing' the dumb-bells in the upward movement.

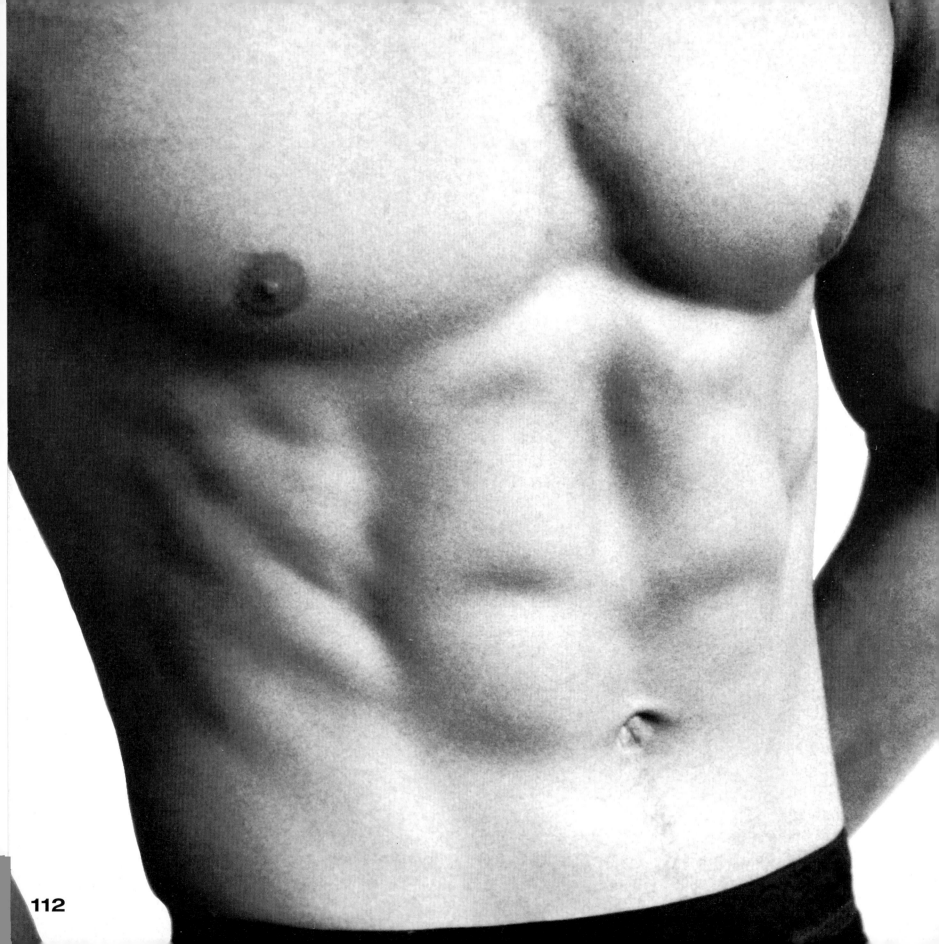

Exercising will help produce the classic 'washboard' stomach. But the real battle for most men is to keep to a minimum the fat layer which easily accumulates over this ridged muscle group!

All exercises should be performed to exhaustion, i.e. to the point at which you cannot achieve another rep.

Rest between sets for only the length of time it has taken you to perform the previous set.

Take a deep breath prior to starting an exercise, then exhale on the exertion and inhale on the recovery. Do not hold your breath – this may dangerously elevate the blood pressure.

SERVICING OF MOVING PARTS ABDOMINALS

Abbreviated to 'abs' for the established gym-goer, you can consider three distinct areas which make up the group: **lower abs**, **obliques** and **upper abs**.

Explore possibilities beyond the exercises shown. Ask for instruction on isolation machines available for specific body parts that you can add into your programme for variety.

There are a few golden rules to effective ab work.

Focus on abs doing the work. It is all too easy to cheat.

The slower you do the exercises the better. This will help with concentration.

10 good repetitions to exhaustion are better than 40 poor ones.

Work on lower abs, followed by obliques, followed by upper abs (the exercises in this section are in this order).

If you do not concentrate properly you will find that the elbows and hips are overriding the effort of your abdominal muscles.

You will find floor exercises more comfortable on a mat, though you may find the 'creep' of your body along them caused by the motion of the exercise irritating.

Hanging knee raise Hang by both hands from a frame, as here, or from a wall-mounted bar, which will usually have step-up blocks nearby so that you do not have to jump to gain your grip.

From certain bars, you may find that at full extension of your body your feet touch the floor. This is not a problem; simply start the exercise from that position.

Raise your knees towards your chest, then lower to the starting position, controlling the downward movement.

Perform the exercise slowly, and avoid, or try to minimise, the swinging motion that will inevitably result in the movement.

As you progress, you may want to try a variation of this exercise, keeping your legs straight as you raise towards your chest. The 'swinging' problem does become worse, though, so you will need extra concentration to overcome this.

Reverse crunch Lie on your back, with your arms at 30 degrees to your body, then raise your legs straight up in the air with feet crossed at the ankles, directly above your lower abs, **1**.

Raise your buttocks off the floor towards the ceiling, **2**. This should be solely achieved as the result of the contraction of the lower abs, and should not be aided by pressure on the floor from your arms, or a kick of the legs.

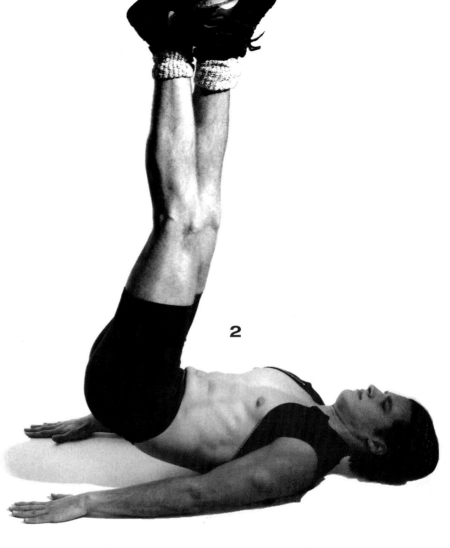

2

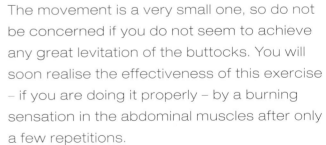

1

The movement is a very small one, so do not be concerned if you do not seem to achieve any great levitation of the buttocks. You will soon realise the effectiveness of this exercise – if you are doing it properly – by a burning sensation in the abdominal muscles after only a few repetitions.

Twisting sit-up Lie on the floor, cradling the back of the head in linked hands. Bring your right leg towards your body so that your upper and lower leg are nearly forming a right angle, then raise your left leg and place your left ankle just below your right knee, **1**.

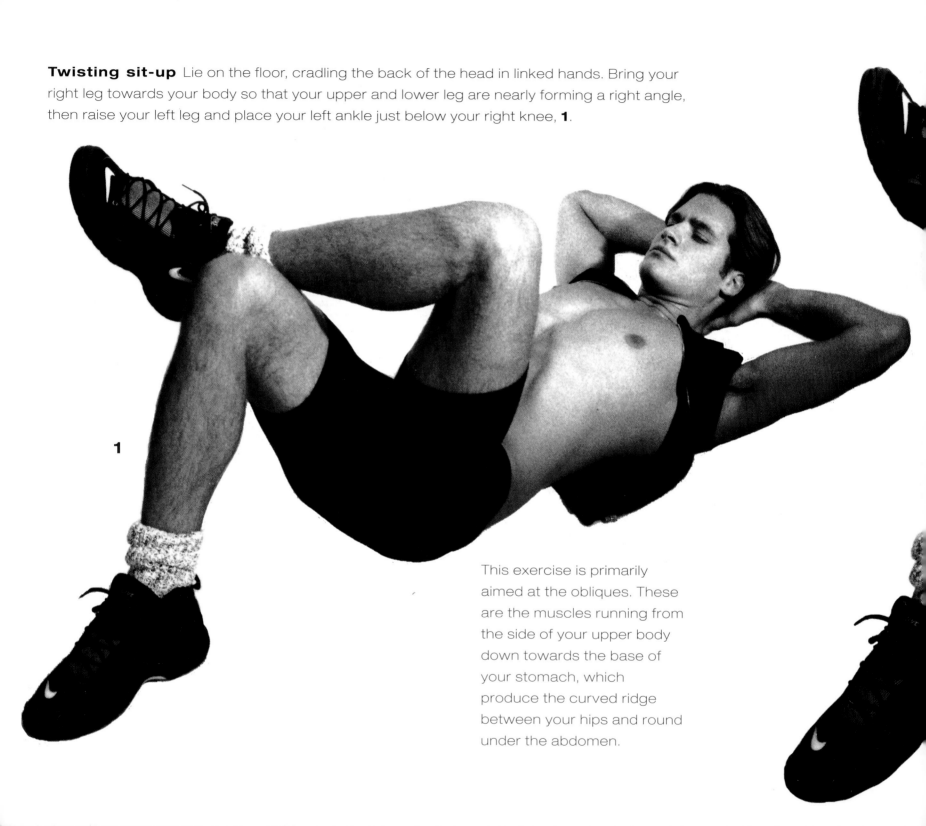

1

This exercise is primarily aimed at the obliques. These are the muscles running from the side of your upper body down towards the base of your stomach, which produce the curved ridge between your hips and round under the abdomen.

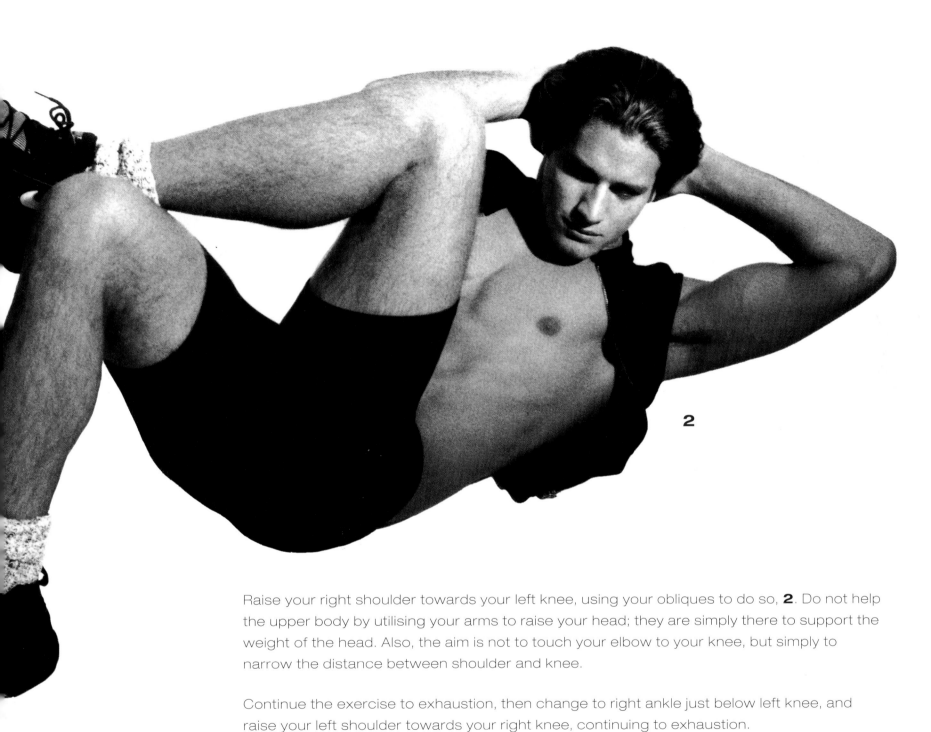

2

Raise your right shoulder towards your left knee, using your obliques to do so, **2**. Do not help the upper body by utilising your arms to raise your head; they are simply there to support the weight of the head. Also, the aim is not to touch your elbow to your knee, but simply to narrow the distance between shoulder and knee.

Continue the exercise to exhaustion, then change to right ankle just below left knee, and raise your left shoulder towards your right knee, continuing to exhaustion.

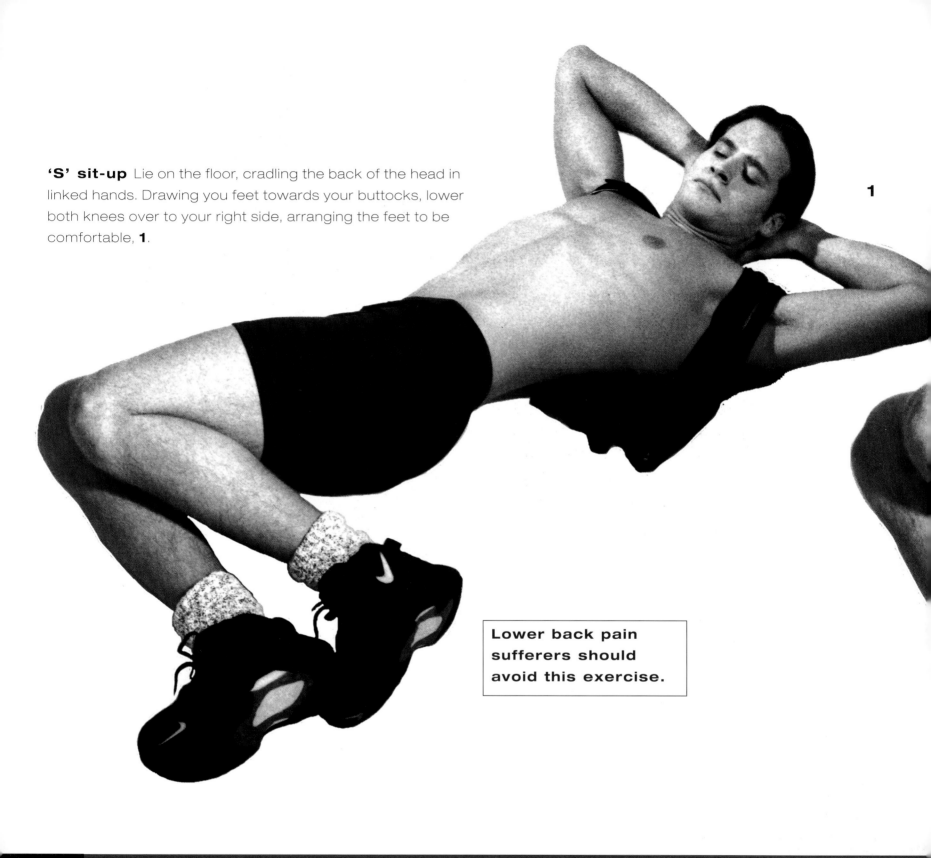

'S' sit-up Lie on the floor, cradling the back of the head in linked hands. Drawing you feet towards your buttocks, lower both knees over to your right side, arranging the feet to be comfortable, **1**.

1

Lower back pain
sufferers should
avoid this exercise.

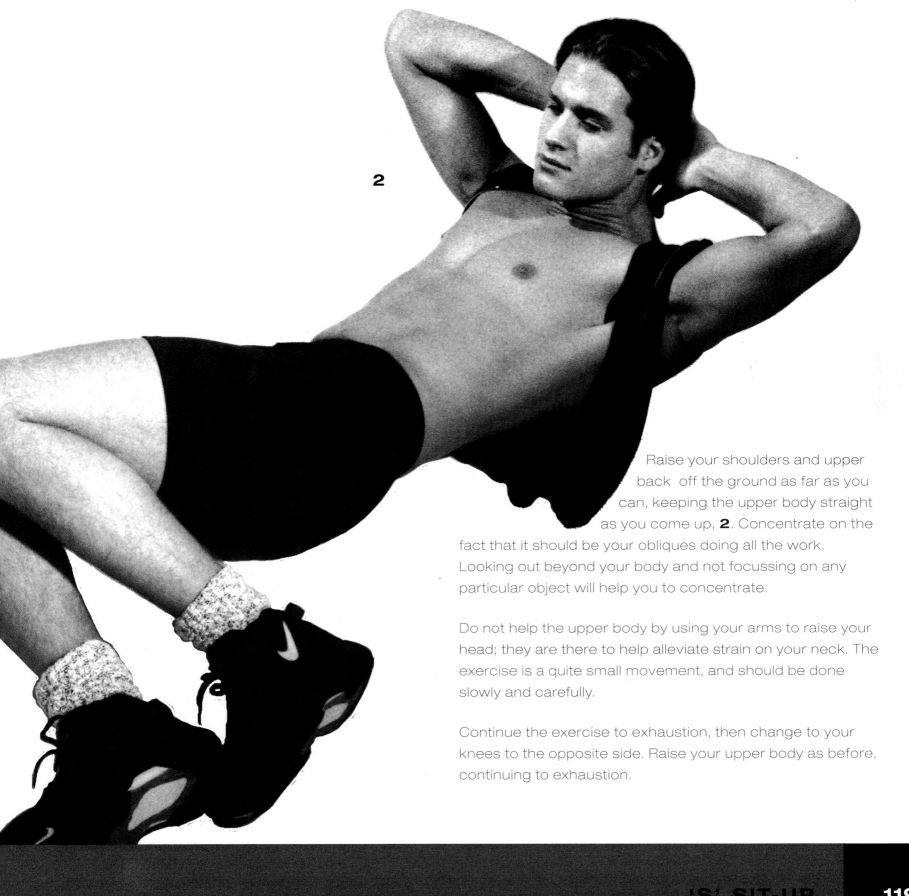

2

Raise your shoulders and upper back off the ground as far as you can, keeping the upper body straight as you come up, **2**. Concentrate on the fact that it should be your obliques doing all the work. Looking out beyond your body and not focussing on any particular object will help you to concentrate.

Do not help the upper body by using your arms to raise your head; they are there to help alleviate strain on your neck. The exercise is a quite small movement, and should be done slowly and carefully.

Continue the exercise to exhaustion, then change to your knees to the opposite side. Raise your upper body as before, continuing to exhaustion.

'S' SIT-UP

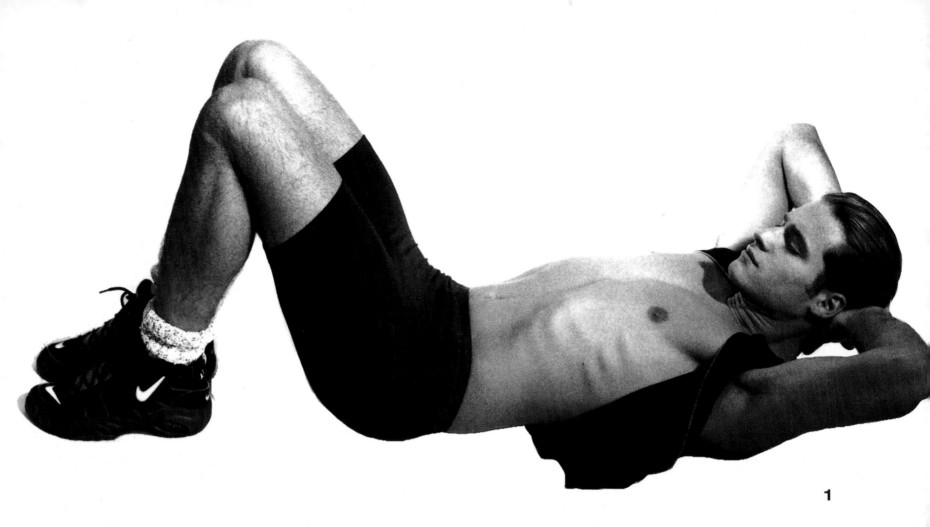

1

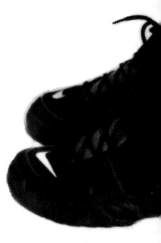

Crunch This is the classic abdominal exercise, but is actually quite difficult to perform effectively.

Lie on the floor with your knees drawn up, and cradle your head in linked hands, **1**.

Concentrating on achieving contraction of the upper abs, curl the upper body up towards your thighs, **2**. Keep the elbows out straight and do not be tempted to bring them round to your ears.

No assistance in the upward movement should be received from the arms pulling your head upwards.

Continue to exhaustion.

This and the next two exercises are **almost** identical exercises – the subtle differences between them should be studied so that you can derive maximum benefit from performing all three.

Key characteristics

Curl up, and 'peel' the vertebrae (the knobbly joints running up your spine) one at a time from the floor.

Focus on your knees as the point towards which you are aiming your head.

2

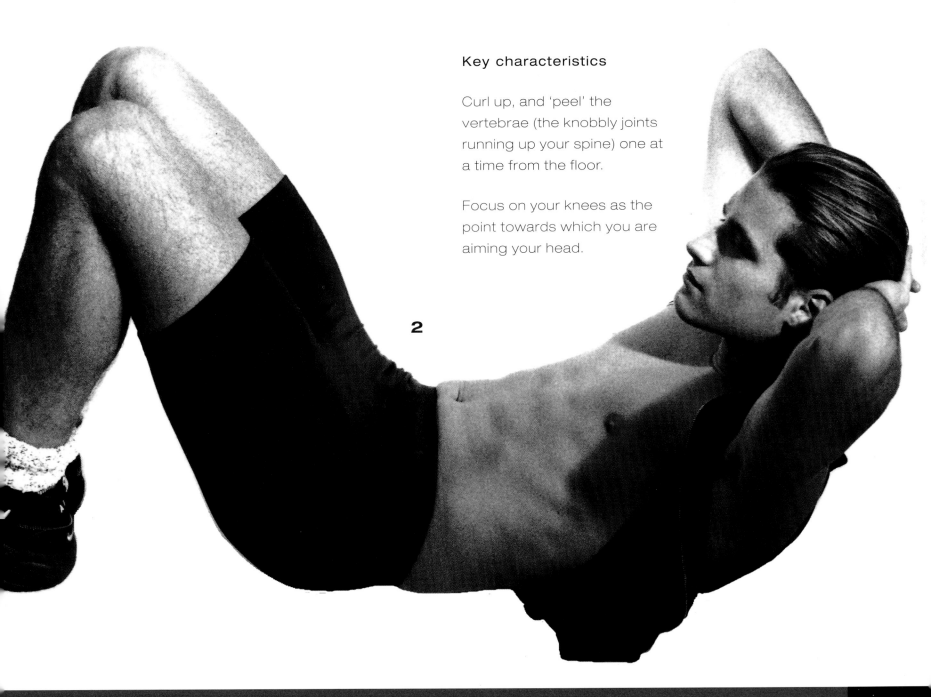

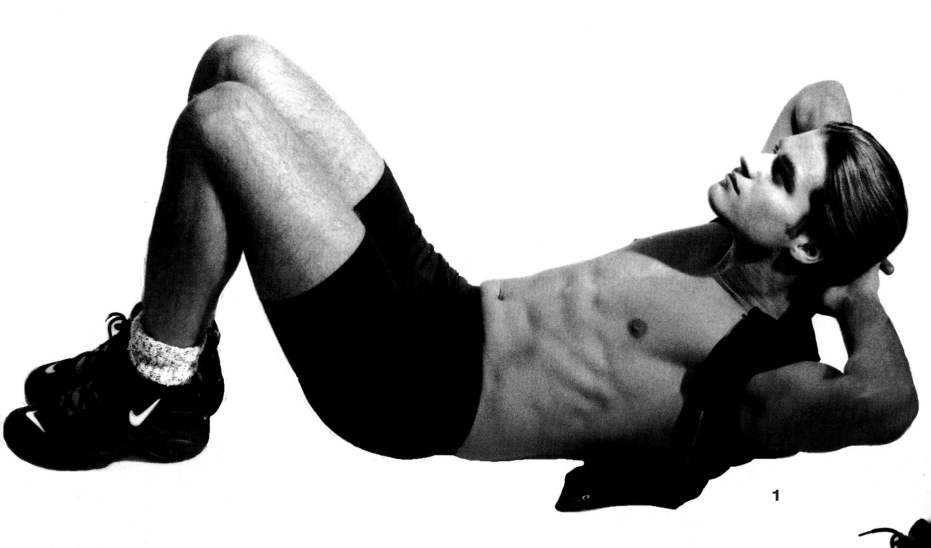

Isolated crunch This is a subtle but distinctly different variety of crunch exercise.

Lie on the floor, knees drawn up, and cradle your head in linked hands as for basic crunch, **1**.

Concentrating on achieving contraction of the upper abs, raise the chest and shoulders upwards in one plane towards the ceiling, **2**. Keep the elbows out straight and do not be tempted to bring them round to your ears, as for basic crunch.

Again, no assistance in the upward movement should be received from the arms pulling your head upwards.

Continue to exhaustion.

This exercise, and the next and the previous exercises, are **almost** identical exercises – the subtle differences between them should be studied so that you can derive maximum benefit from performing all three.

Key characteristics

Keep your head and shoulders back. The exercise is made more difficult than the simple crunch by the fact that the head and shoulders are further from the hips, which act as the fulcrum for the pivot.

Focus on the ceiling as the point towards which you are aiming your head.

2

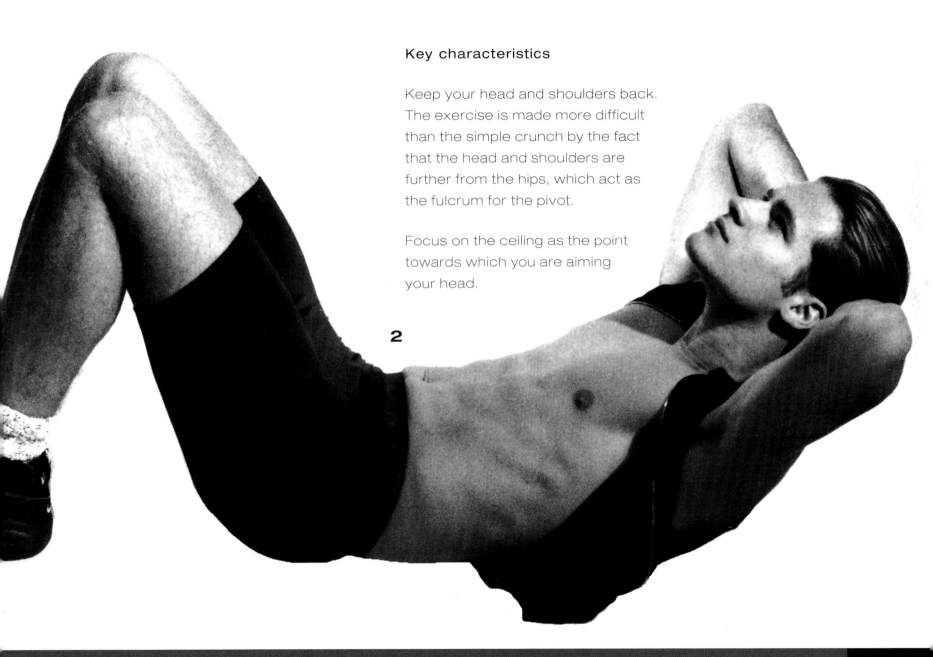

Double crunch Essentially this is a two-stage version of the basic crunch. The theory is that when you have 'crunched' you can always 'crunch' a little more.

Lie on the floor, knees drawn up, and cradle your head in linked hands as for basic crunch, **1**.

Concentrating on achieving contraction of the upper abs, curl your upper body up towards your thighs, as for basic crunch, **2**. Keep the elbows out straight and do not be tempted to bring them round to your ears, as for basic crunch.

Again, no assistance in the upward movement should be received from the arms pulling your head upwards.

Immediately following the first crunch effort – and this requires both concentration and determination – contract the abdominal muscles even further, **3**.

Continue to exhaustion.

Be especially vigilant about not using the arms for an extra 'push' to achieve this, and do not cheat by only putting in a half-effort in the initial crunch.

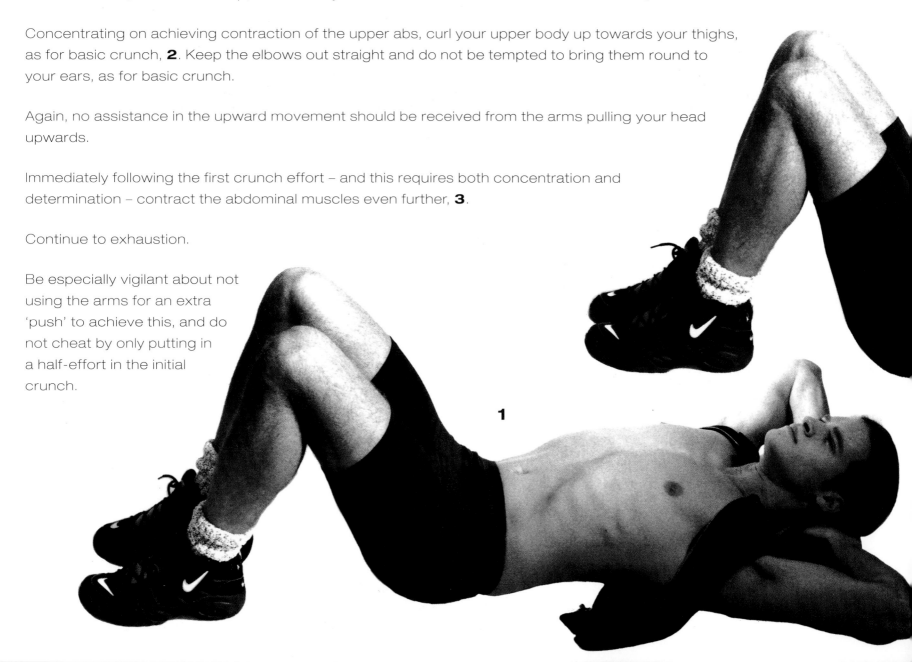

1

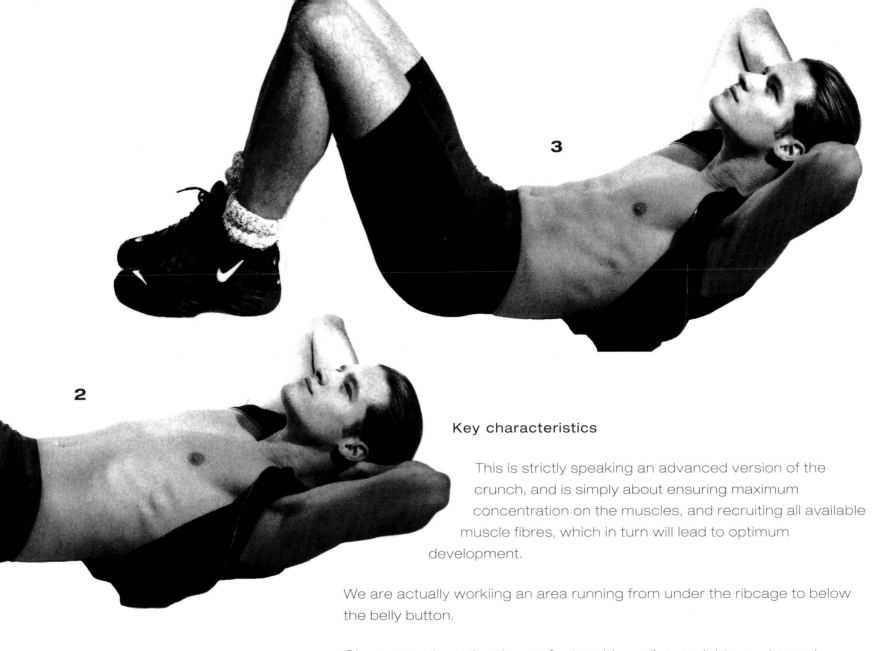

3

2

Key characteristics

This is strictly speaking an advanced version of the crunch, and is simply about ensuring maximum concentration on the muscles, and recruiting all available muscle fibres, which in turn will lead to optimum development.

We are actually workiing an area running from under the ribcage to below the belly button.

Given our automotive theme, for 'washboard' you might care to read radiator grill, for a more up-to-date analogy.

> This and the previous two exercises are **almost** identical exercises – the subtle differences between them should be studied so that you can derive maximum benefit from performing all three.

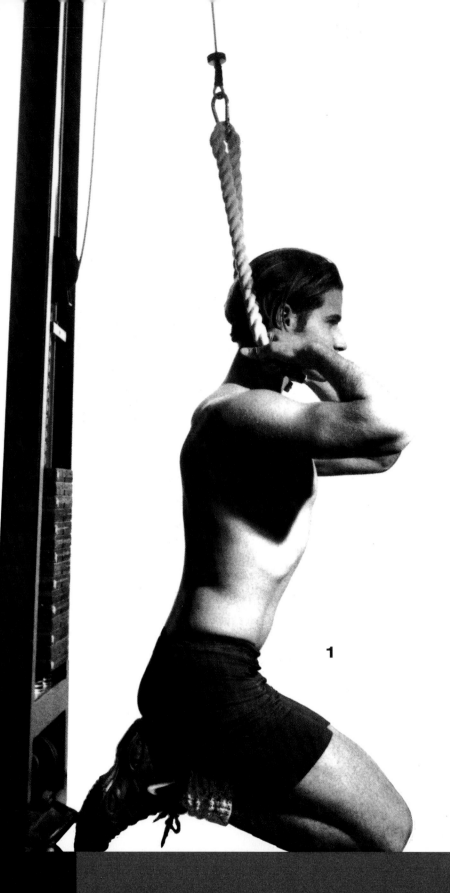

Pulley crunch This is the only exercise in this section which requires a machine; it provides a resistance to the movement performed.

Attach the rope fitting to the upper pulley of one end of a cable machine, and set a suitable weight on the weight rack. Be careful when doing this exercise for the first time that you are not over ambitious with the amount of weight – a light weight will suffice if your technique is good.

Kneel in front of the cable machine, holding the two ends of the rope either side of your head at neck level, **1**. There are generally either knots in the rope at the ends, or grips as on bicycle handlebars, which you can grasp.

1

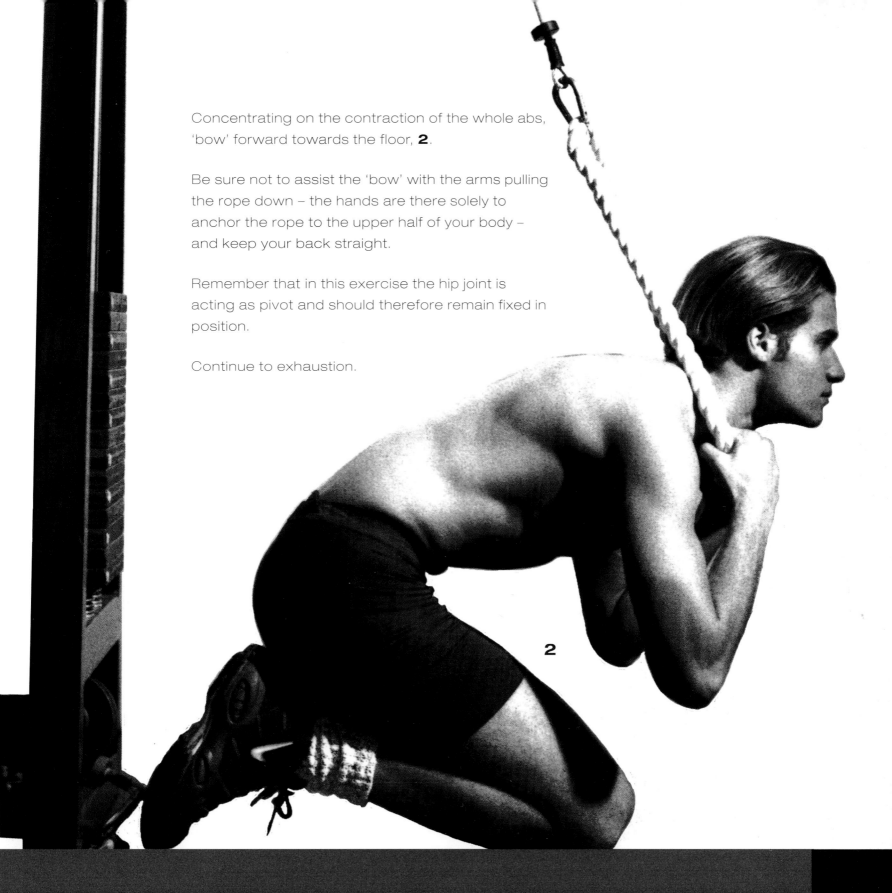

Concentrating on the contraction of the whole abs, 'bow' forward towards the floor, **2**.

Be sure not to assist the 'bow' with the arms pulling the rope down – the hands are there solely to anchor the rope to the upper half of your body – and keep your back straight.

Remember that in this exercise the hip joint is acting as pivot and should therefore remain fixed in position.

Continue to exhaustion.

2

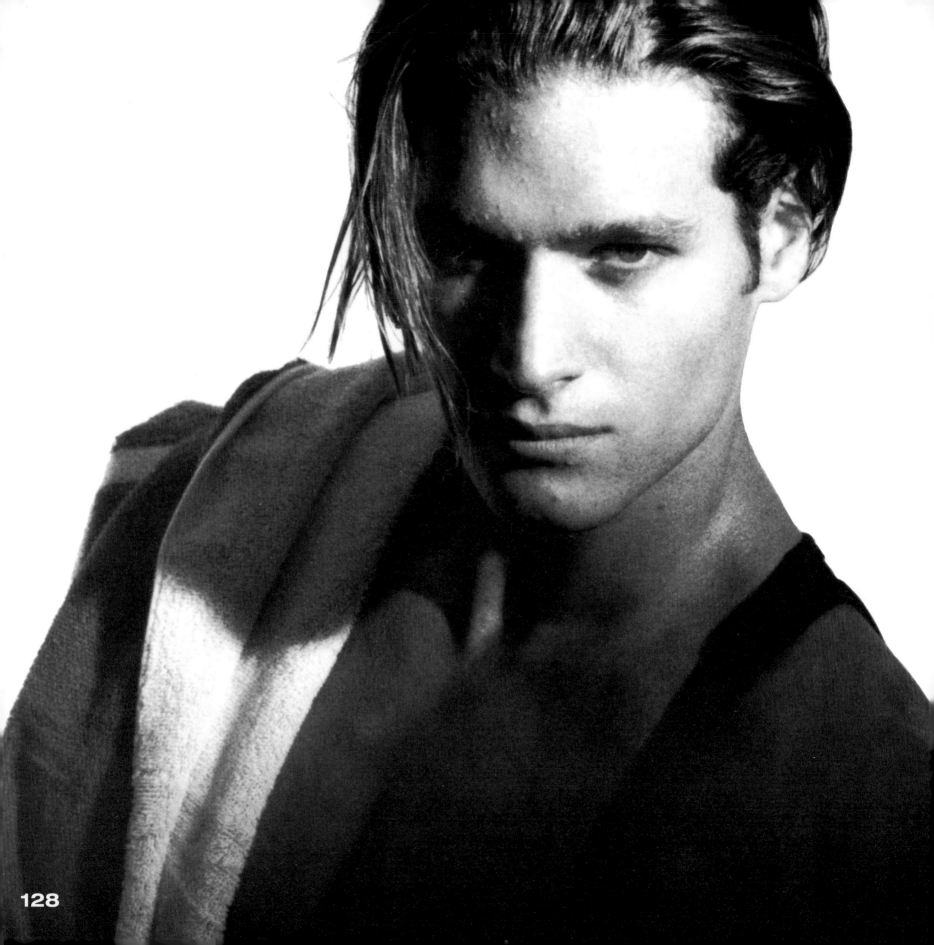

You've finished your workout and think you're finished, but stopping dead is like taking a hot engine and plunging it in a bucket of cold water – damage could result.

PARKING

Bring your body back to normal running speed by giving yourself enough time to decelerate naturally – and even relax.

Section essentials

Never finish a workout without a cool-down.

Slow yourself down first with reverse cardio-vascular exercise.

Rest for a period after reverse cardio-vascular exercise – your body should be encouraged to cool down.

Hold the cool-down exercise positions (pages 128-137) for a minimum count of fifteen as this will also encourage your body to cool down. Try to hold for longer if possible.

If you choose to skip reverse cardio-vascular work at the gym, because you will cycle or run home, do not skip your stretch exercises.

Breathe freely and deeply during the whole of your cool-down.

Do not hold your breath during any exercise – breathe normally.

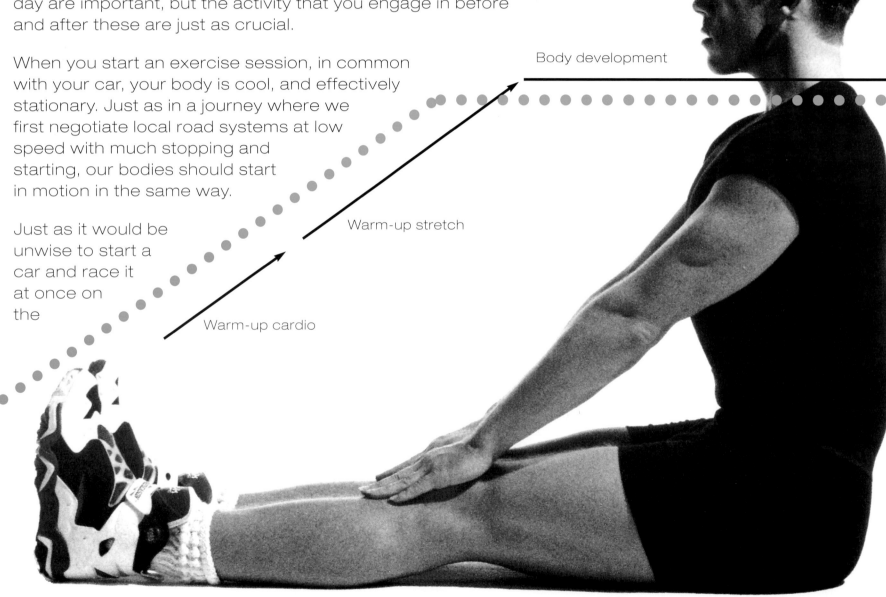

HILL RACING

The secret of a good workout is its structure. The exercises that you choose to perform for the development of your body on a certain day are important, but the activity that you engage in before and after these are just as crucial.

When you start an exercise session, in common with your car, your body is cool, and effectively stationary. Just as in a journey where we first negotiate local road systems at low speed with much stopping and starting, our bodies should start in motion in the same way.

Just as it would be unwise to start a car and race it at once on the

Body development

Warm-up stretch

Warm-up cardio

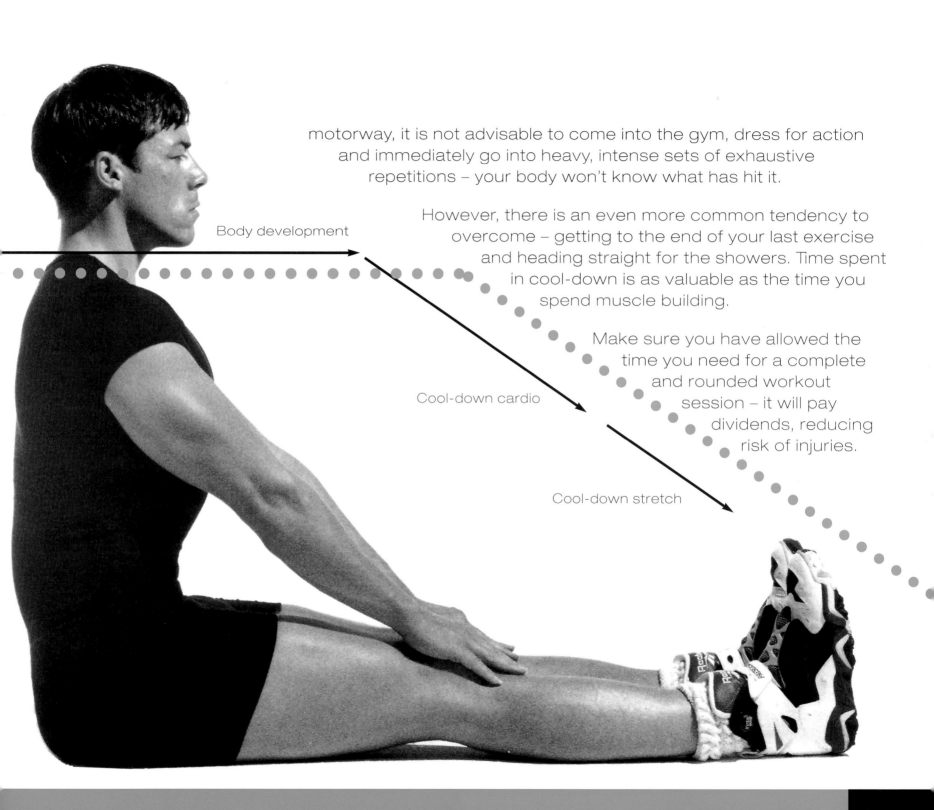

motorway, it is not advisable to come into the gym, dress for action and immediately go into heavy, intense sets of exhaustive repetitions – your body won't know what has hit it.

However, there is an even more common tendency to overcome – getting to the end of your last exercise and heading straight for the showers. Time spent in cool-down is as valuable as the time you spend muscle building.

Make sure you have allowed the time you need for a complete and rounded workout session – it will pay dividends, reducing risk of injuries.

Body development

Cool-down cardio

Cool-down stretch

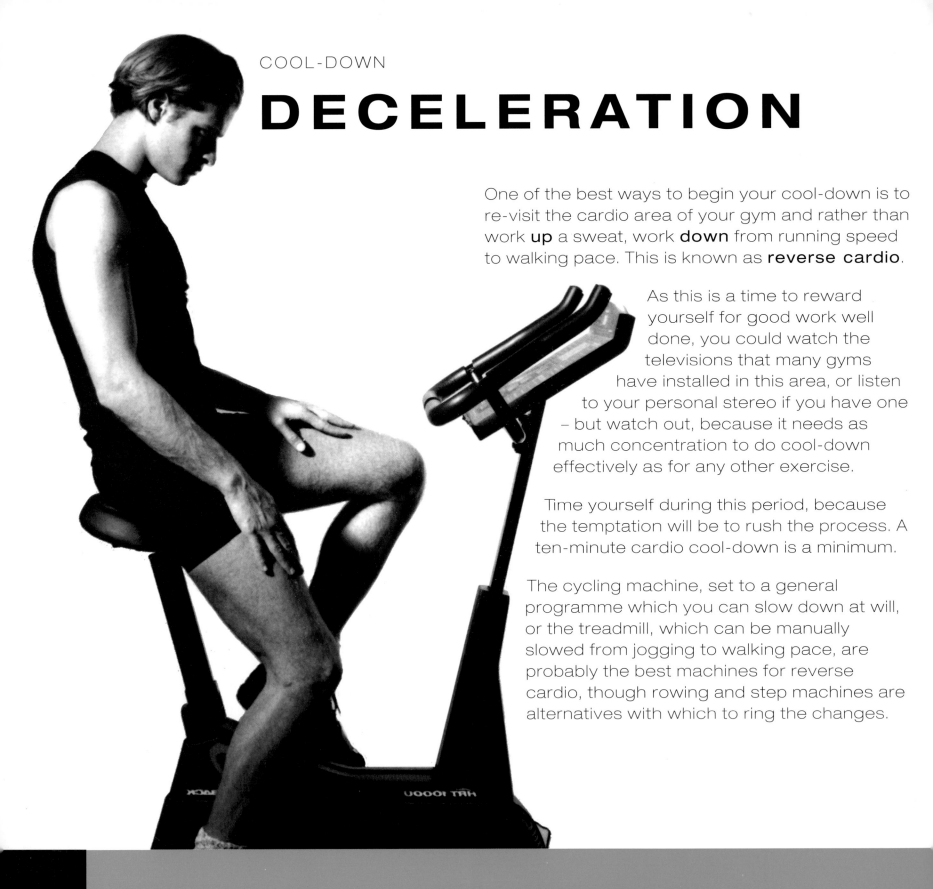

COOL-DOWN

DECELERATION

One of the best ways to begin your cool-down is to re-visit the cardio area of your gym and rather than work **up** a sweat, work **down** from running speed to walking pace. This is known as **reverse cardio**.

As this is a time to reward yourself for good work well done, you could watch the televisions that many gyms have installed in this area, or listen to your personal stereo if you have one – but watch out, because it needs as much concentration to do cool-down effectively as for any other exercise.

Time yourself during this period, because the temptation will be to rush the process. A ten-minute cardio cool-down is a minimum.

The cycling machine, set to a general programme which you can slow down at will, or the treadmill, which can be manually slowed from jogging to walking pace, are probably the best machines for reverse cardio, though rowing and step machines are alternatives with which to ring the changes.

A less widely-practised alternative or additional method of cool-down, is **reprise training**.

When your muscles have been worked intensively it is often possible for them to feel as if they are knotted in your body. They are quite literally 'pumped-up', being full of blood.

Freeing them again is simply a matter of going through the motions of all the exercises you have performed for the particular body parts of the day in question – but this time without weights. Reprise training will aid venous return, that is, the blood returning to vital organs where it is best used at rest.

This type of cool-down can be extremely effective in regaining a full range of motion after intensive exercise. It is one of the best-kept secrets of professional sportsmen and women.

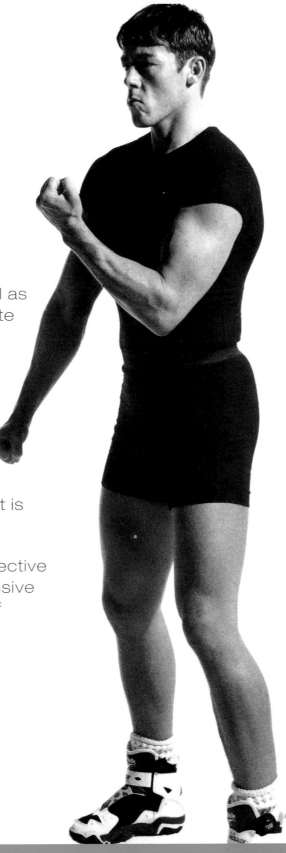

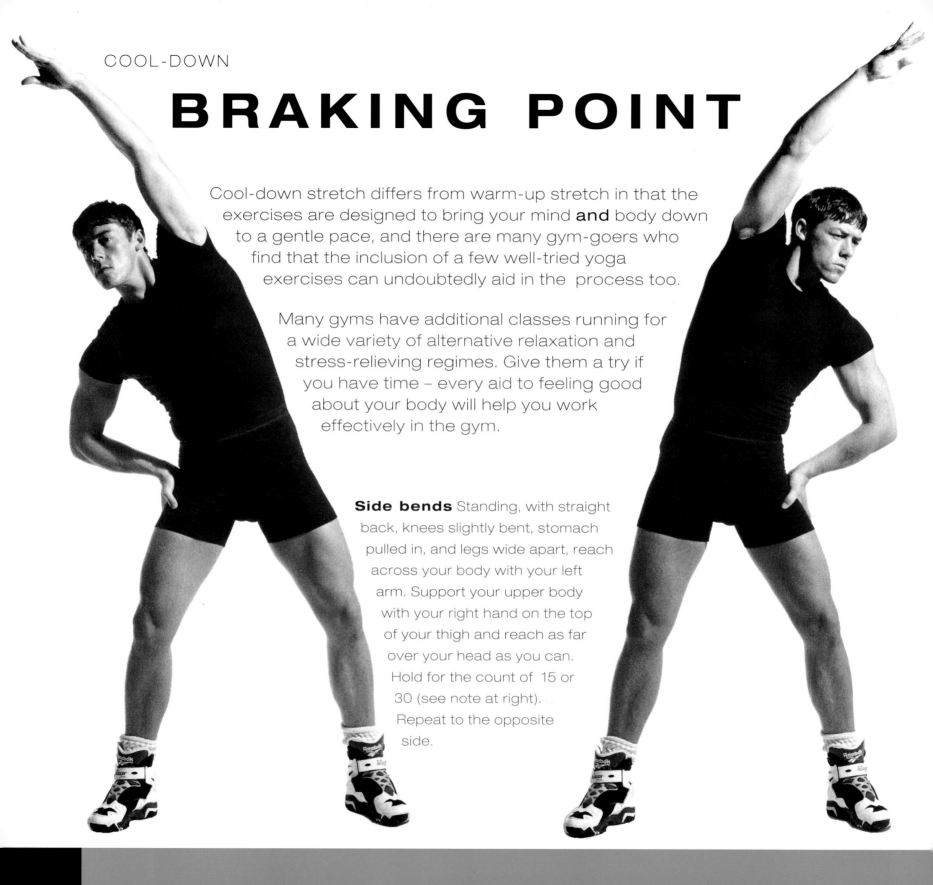

BRAKING POINT

Cool-down stretch differs from warm-up stretch in that the exercises are designed to bring your mind **and** body down to a gentle pace, and there are many gym-goers who find that the inclusion of a few well-tried yoga exercises can undoubtedly aid in the process too.

Many gyms have additional classes running for a wide variety of alternative relaxation and stress-relieving regimes. Give them a try if you have time – every aid to feeling good about your body will help you work effectively in the gym.

Side bends Standing, with straight back, knees slightly bent, stomach pulled in, and legs wide apart, reach across your body with your left arm. Support your upper body with your right hand on the top of your thigh and reach as far over your head as you can. Hold for the count of 15 or 30 (see note at right). Repeat to the opposite side.

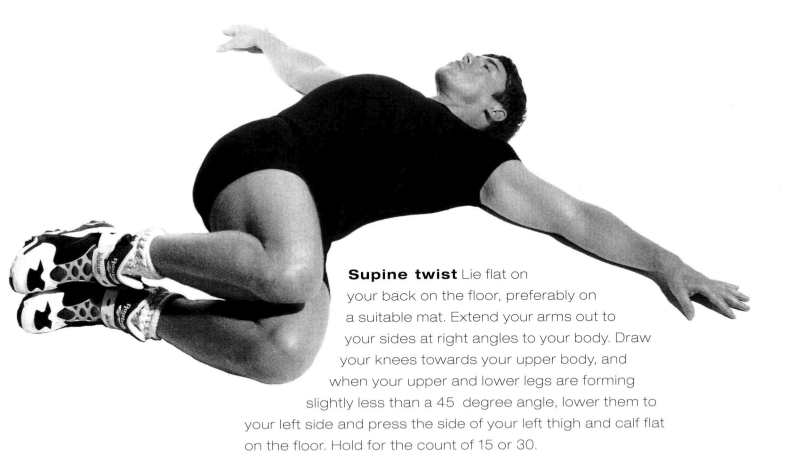

Supine twist Lie flat on
your back on the floor, preferably on
a suitable mat. Extend your arms out to
your sides at right angles to your body. Draw
your knees towards your upper body, and
when your upper and lower legs are forming
slightly less than a 45 degree angle, lower them to
your left side and press the side of your left thigh and calf flat
on the floor. Hold for the count of 15 or 30.

Repeat, swinging your legs to the right.

**How long to hold
the stretch**

A count of 15
seconds *maintains*
the level of flexibility
in the muscles

A count of at
least 30
seconds
develops the
level of flexibility
in the muscles

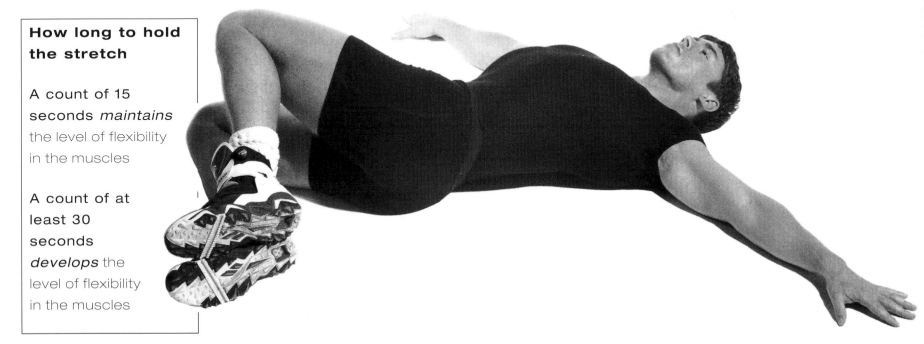

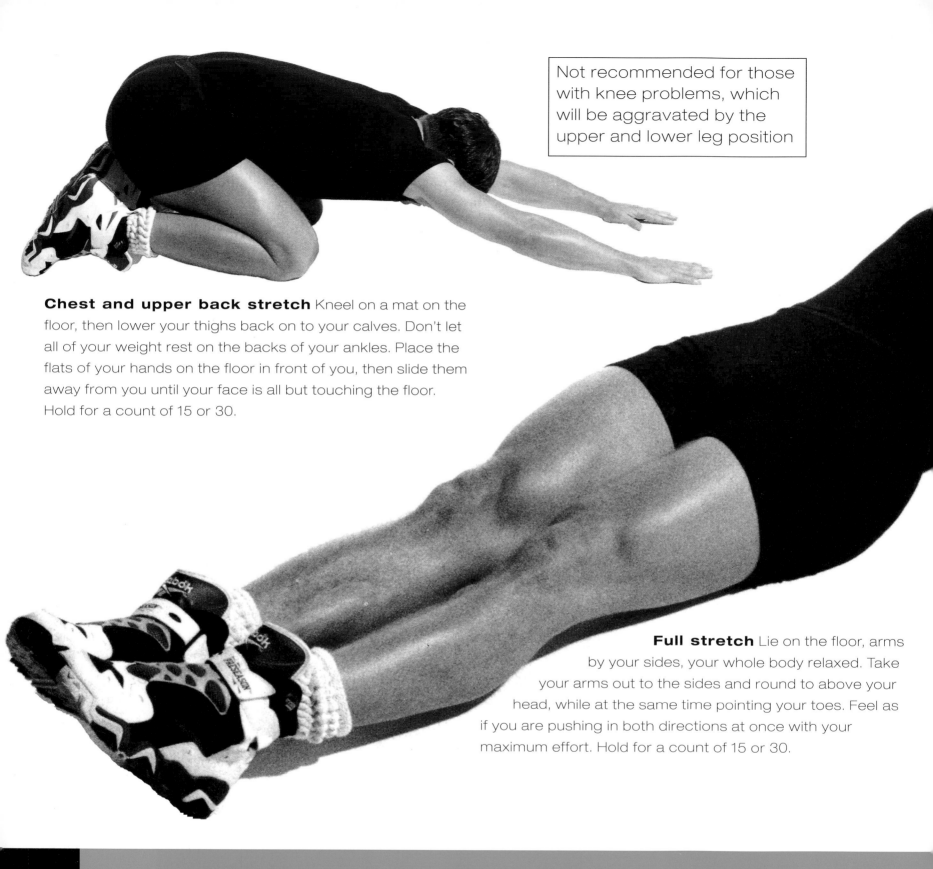

Not recommended for those with knee problems, which will be aggravated by the upper and lower leg position

Chest and upper back stretch Kneel on a mat on the floor, then lower your thighs back on to your calves. Don't let all of your weight rest on the backs of your ankles. Place the flats of your hands on the floor in front of you, then slide them away from you until your face is all but touching the floor. Hold for a count of 15 or 30.

Full stretch Lie on the floor, arms by your sides, your whole body relaxed. Take your arms out to the sides and round to above your head, while at the same time pointing your toes. Feel as if you are pushing in both directions at once with your maximum effort. Hold for a count of 15 or 30.

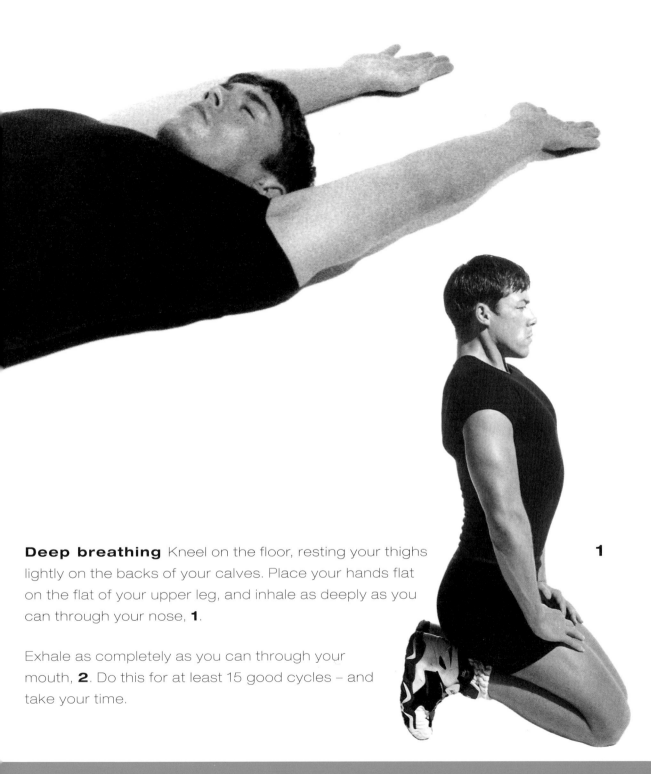

Okay – *now* you can head for the showers.

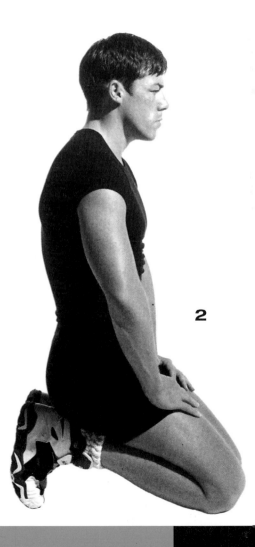

Deep breathing Kneel on the floor, resting your thighs lightly on the backs of your calves. Place your hands flat on the flat of your upper leg, and inhale as deeply as you can through your nose, **1**.

Exhale as completely as you can through your mouth, **2**. Do this for at least 15 good cycles – and take your time.

1

2

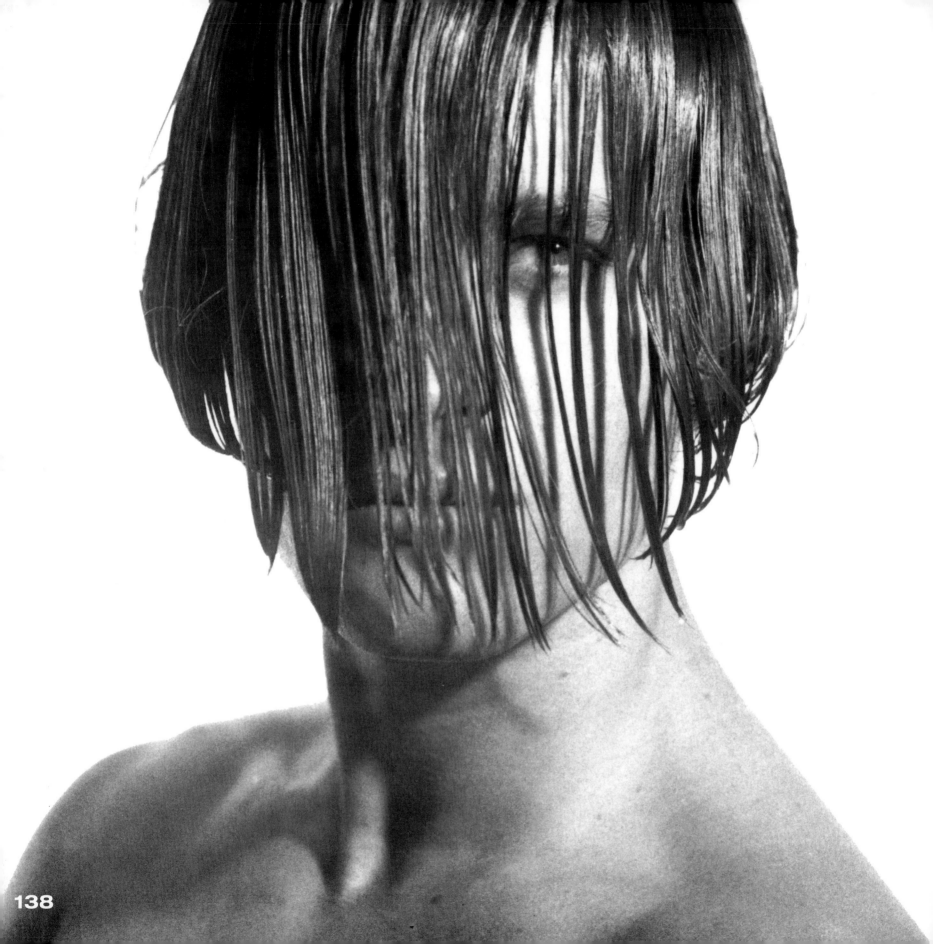

You may be out of the workshop, but now is time to come to terms with the actual bodywork. You're about to show the world what you've made of yourself – so take time over your valetting.

CARE OF BODYWORK

A simple maintenance routine will enhance your training results.

FINISHES

If you've gone all-out in the gym to get your physique in top condition, you really also ought to devote some time to the outer layer – which is, after all, what *others* actually see.

Regular skin maintenance can make a very real difference to the toll that time takes on your physical appearance. It need not take long, once you know the basic rules, to get into the habit of performing an effective skin routine that suits you.

Just like the car-wash, there are three stages to a gleaming finish: **wash**, **dry** and **polish**. You'll also be aware that there are different levels at the car-wash, and that you get what you pay for. Don't scrimp on the time you take, or the money you spend – or you'll get the same result you get with your car.

Taking too much time over your appearance used to be considered a sure sign of vanity. Nowadays, even the most aggressively masculine type will acknowledge the value of a basic moisturiser or a good skin cleanser. Once again of course, sports professionals who have driven their bodies to the edge have known the benefits for years. All-round health for them is always reflected in performance.

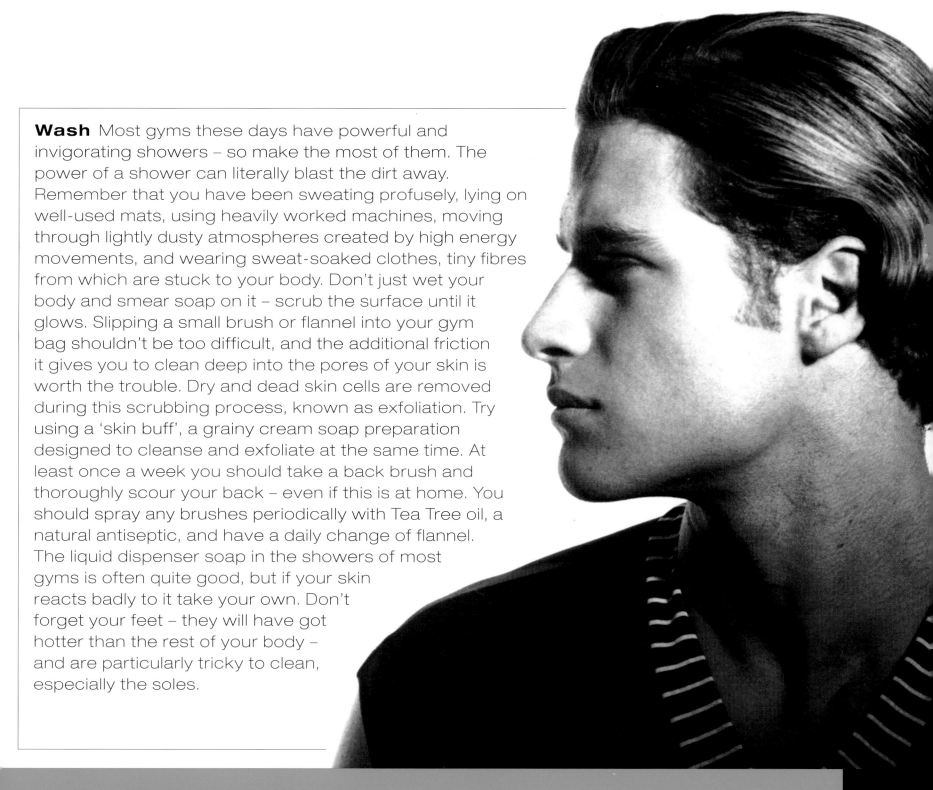

Wash Most gyms these days have powerful and invigorating showers – so make the most of them. The power of a shower can literally blast the dirt away. Remember that you have been sweating profusely, lying on well-used mats, using heavily worked machines, moving through lightly dusty atmospheres created by high energy movements, and wearing sweat-soaked clothes, tiny fibres from which are stuck to your body. Don't just wet your body and smear soap on it – scrub the surface until it glows. Slipping a small brush or flannel into your gym bag shouldn't be too difficult, and the additional friction it gives you to clean deep into the pores of your skin is worth the trouble. Dry and dead skin cells are removed during this scrubbing process, known as exfoliation. Try using a 'skin buff', a grainy cream soap preparation designed to cleanse and exfoliate at the same time. At least once a week you should take a back brush and thoroughly scour your back – even if this is at home. You should spray any brushes periodically with Tea Tree oil, a natural antiseptic, and have a daily change of flannel. The liquid dispenser soap in the showers of most gyms is often quite good, but if your skin reacts badly to it take your own. Don't forget your feet – they will have got hotter than the rest of your body – and are particularly tricky to clean, especially the soles.

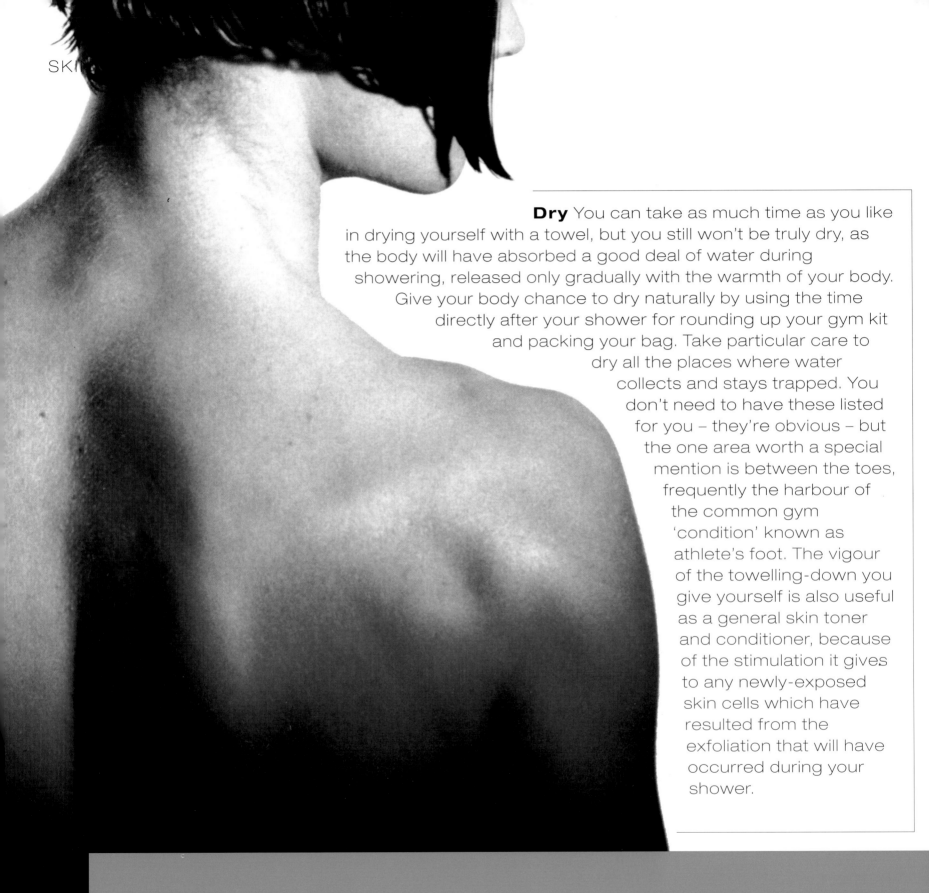

Dry You can take as much time as you like in drying yourself with a towel, but you still won't be truly dry, as the body will have absorbed a good deal of water during showering, released only gradually with the warmth of your body. Give your body chance to dry naturally by using the time directly after your shower for rounding up your gym kit and packing your bag. Take particular care to dry all the places where water collects and stays trapped. You don't need to have these listed for you – they're obvious – but the one area worth a special mention is between the toes, frequently the harbour of the common gym 'condition' known as athlete's foot. The vigour of the towelling-down you give yourself is also useful as a general skin toner and conditioner, because of the stimulation it gives to any newly-exposed skin cells which have resulted from the exfoliation that will have occurred during your shower.

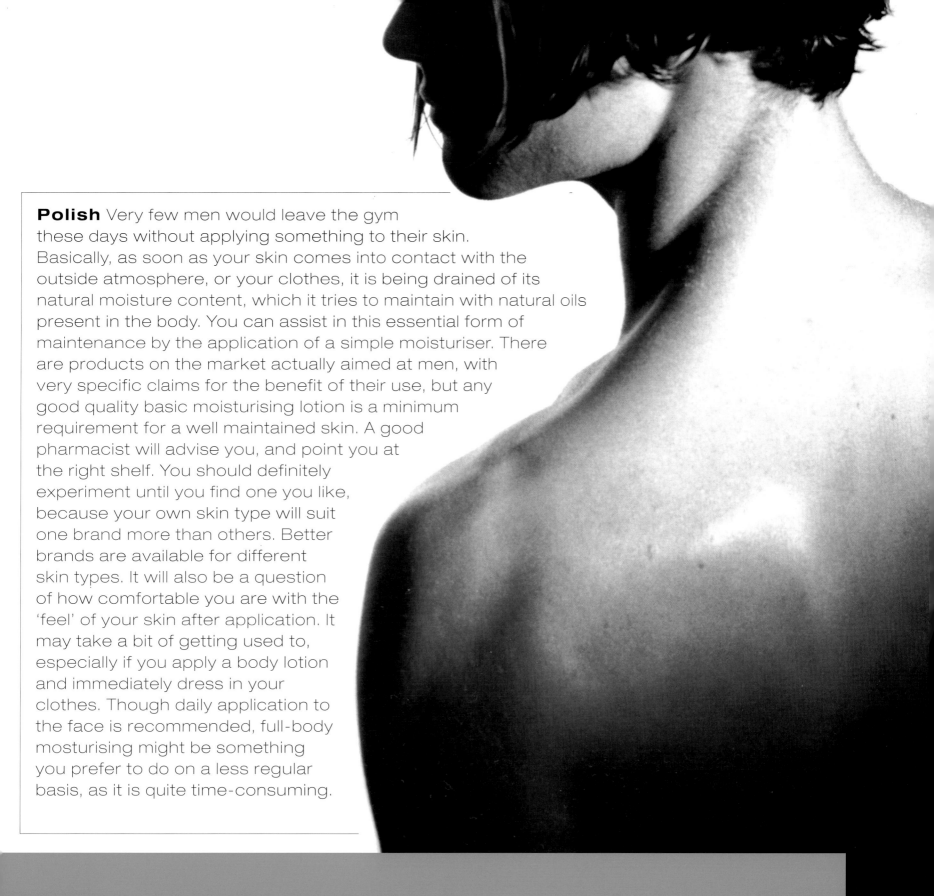

Polish Very few men would leave the gym these days without applying something to their skin. Basically, as soon as your skin comes into contact with the outside atmosphere, or your clothes, it is being drained of its natural moisture content, which it tries to maintain with natural oils present in the body. You can assist in this essential form of maintenance by the application of a simple moisturiser. There are products on the market actually aimed at men, with very specific claims for the benefit of their use, but any good quality basic moisturising lotion is a minimum requirement for a well maintained skin. A good pharmacist will advise you, and point you at the right shelf. You should definitely experiment until you find one you like, because your own skin type will suit one brand more than others. Better brands are available for different skin types. It will also be a question of how comfortable you are with the 'feel' of your skin after application. It may take a bit of getting used to, especially if you apply a body lotion and immediately dress in your clothes. Though daily application to the face is recommended, full-body mosturising might be something you prefer to do on a less regular basis, as it is quite time-consuming.

UPHOLSTERY

As has already been stated in connection with your body, you have to work with what you've got, and your hair is no exception to this simple rule. Though you may choose to go through life wishing you had someone else's hair, it is probably far better for your own health and sanity to simply try to do what is best for the particular hand – or head of hair – you've been dealt.

Whether you have a lot or a little, one thing is sure; well cut and cared for hair has its own appeal. Find a barber or hairdresser you like and trust, and try to visit them once a month.

Avoid telling him or her what to do. They, like mechanics, have had years of training, and have seen every type and texture going.

The condition of your hair will also make a huge difference to how it looks, and all too frequently the most simple steps to healthy hair maintenance are rushed or ignored completely in daily gym routine.

Working out can often mean that you are washing your hair more than once a day. The hair has a natural balance of moisture and natural oils which washing can remove.

For the gym, a few sensible guidelines should therefore be observed:

• Choose your shampoo with care, and make sure it suits your particular hair type. You want one that cleanses gently, and yet doesn't strip your hair of its essential moisture.

• In addition to the normal categories of dry, normal and oily, shampoos frequently make reference to protein content. These are particularly useful to gym-goers, because the protein adds a protective layer to make the hair stronger and more manageable.

• You should use as little shampoo as possible, and spend the maximum you can afford on it. A single shampooing, a gentle conditioning scalp massage, and a thorough rinse will be sufficient, despite what it says on the bottle.

• In general, the combination liquid soap and shampoo in the dispensers at gyms should not be used regularly on your hair, as it will be of a very general suitability and probably dry out your hair unduly.

• If you shampoo daily, you don't need to use a conditioner every time you wash your hair.

• Invest in good quality combs and brushes, and don't use anything that feels as if it is tearing your hair out.

• Use a brush when using a hair dryer, as this will mean the air is not blowing directly on the scalp or hair.

Stay away from combined shampoo and conditioner products – ask any hairdresser why!

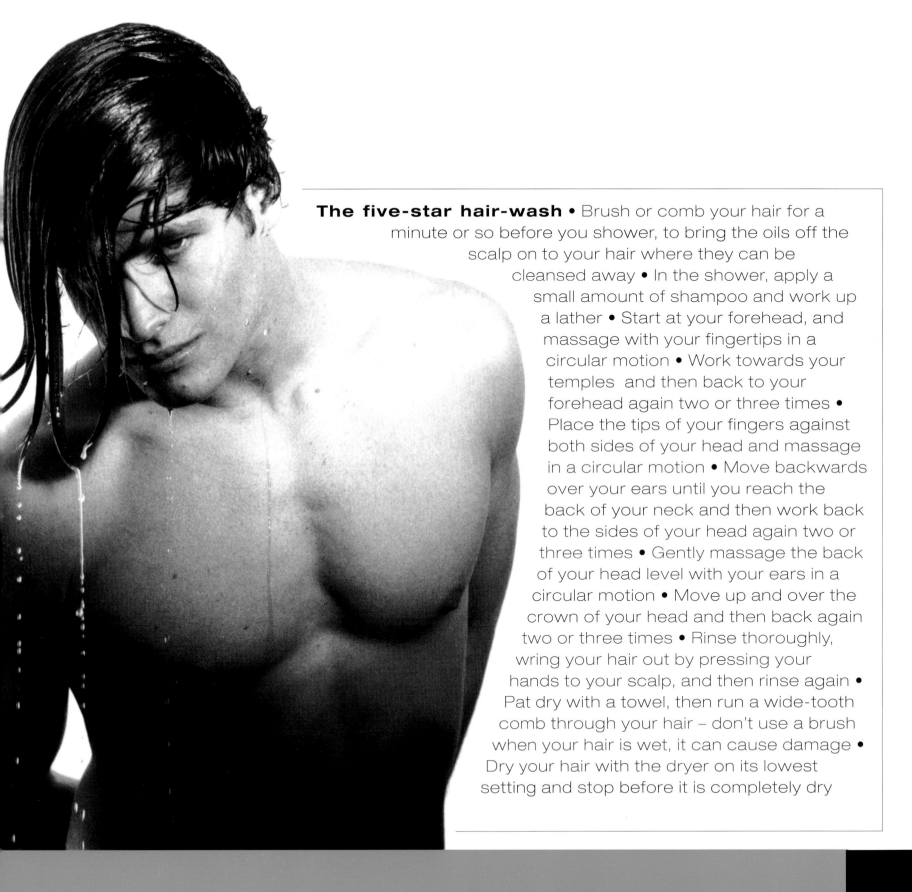

The five-star hair-wash • Brush or comb your hair for a minute or so before you shower, to bring the oils off the scalp on to your hair where they can be cleansed away • In the shower, apply a small amount of shampoo and work up a lather • Start at your forehead, and massage with your fingertips in a circular motion • Work towards your temples and then back to your forehead again two or three times • Place the tips of your fingers against both sides of your head and massage in a circular motion • Move backwards over your ears until you reach the back of your neck and then work back to the sides of your head again two or three times • Gently massage the back of your head level with your ears in a circular motion • Move up and over the crown of your head and then back again two or three times • Rinse thoroughly, wring your hair out by pressing your hands to your scalp, and then rinse again • Pat dry with a towel, then run a wide-tooth comb through your hair – don't use a brush when your hair is wet, it can cause damage • Dry your hair with the dryer on its lowest setting and stop before it is completely dry

Hair is not only, of course, confined to the top of men's heads. As much attention needs to be given to facial hair and its treatment, since the procedure for its maintenance is inextricably linked to the care of the skin.

Dragging a blade across the surface of the face seems as mad as taking a coin to the side of a car, yet it is done daily.

Softening the skin prior to this attack, and then soothing it afterwards, should be considered as important procedures for the preservation of the perfect body finish.

The closest shave is undoubtedly achieved in the wet, warm and steam-filled atmosphere of a shower, as your facial hair will be softened to the maximum. But you will find that most gyms will not permit shaving in the shower area, so this may be a method you can only use at home.

Experiment with the many foams and gels available for your preferred brand. Irritation after shaving may well be from the product you use rather than from shaving itself.

If you have a particularly heavy beard, a second shave might be needed. Two light shaves are better for your skin than one heavy one.

Do not underestimate the importance of good light to shave by. You'll have fewer accidents, and miss less stubble.

The five-star basin shave • Run a basin of hot water • Immerse your facecloth, wring it lightly, then apply it flat to your face for ten seconds • Massage your face with your hands, moving from forehead to neck • Splash your face five times from the basin • Rub a bar of glycerine soap over your beard (the clear kind you can get from good chemists) • Wash your face with a facecloth, working against the grain of your beard • Rinse off the lather made with the cloth by again splashing your face five times • Rub your beard with the soap bar again and work up a lather with your facecloth, remembering to work against the grain of your beard as before • Run hot water on a shaving brush and work up the lather to an even thicker one, or apply your preferred shaving gel or foam • Shave, **going with the grain of your beard**, working methodically around your face from under one ear round past your mouth and ending at the other ear, then working back under your chin and on your neck, with your head up, to where you started • Rinse off your face with five hot splashes of water, then five cold • Pat your face dry with a towel – a non-piled cotton towel like a barber would use is best • Apply a moisturiser

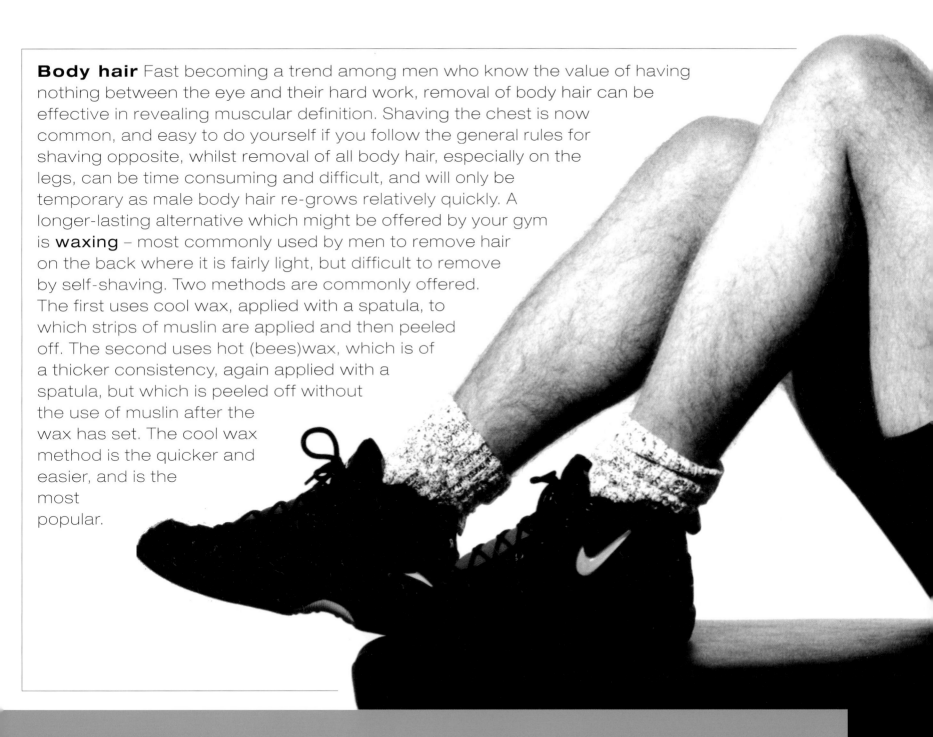

Body hair Fast becoming a trend among men who know the value of having nothing between the eye and their hard work, removal of body hair can be effective in revealing muscular definition. Shaving the chest is now common, and easy to do yourself if you follow the general rules for shaving opposite, whilst removal of all body hair, especially on the legs, can be time consuming and difficult, and will only be temporary as male body hair re-grows relatively quickly. A longer-lasting alternative which might be offered by your gym is **waxing** – most commonly used by men to remove hair on the back where it is fairly light, but difficult to remove by self-shaving. Two methods are commonly offered. The first uses cool wax, applied with a spatula, to which strips of muslin are applied and then peeled off. The second uses hot (bees)wax, which is of a thicker consistency, again applied with a spatula, but which is peeled off without the use of muslin after the wax has set. The cool wax method is the quicker and easier, and is the most popular.

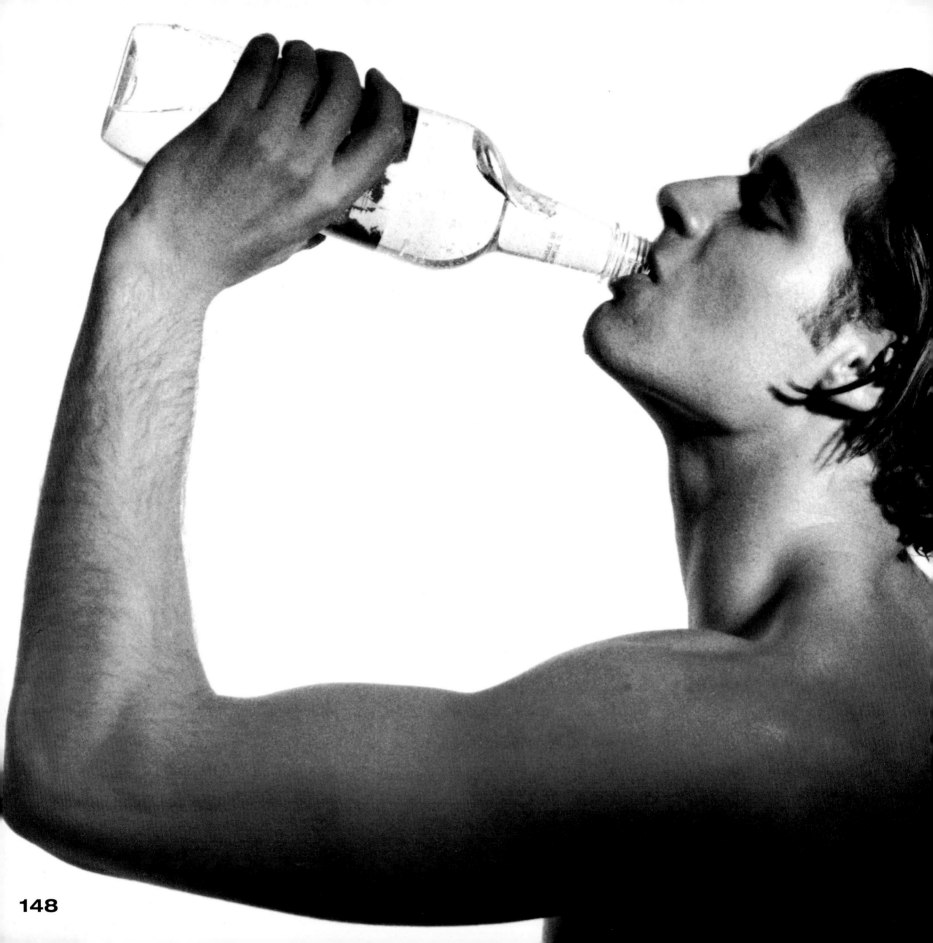

Cars don't run on air and neither do we – but of the wider choice of fuels on offer to the human engine, not all are suitable for consumption by those in pursuit of a well-tuned body.

FUELS & LUBRICANTS

Keeping the motor running smoothly also requires effective additives.

HIGH OCTANE

There won't be many surprises in the next few pages of this book. Health education has made it clear to all of us how our eating habits can affect our well-being, and gym-goers are more aware than most when they are consuming a less-than-healthy meal.

Yet few people really understand the importance of diet in their training programme. Most men assume that it is the amount of work they put in at the gym in terms of reps and sets, and workout frequency, that will result in progress, when in fact up to half of any monitorable change in their bodies will be attributable to nutritional habits.

Four key factors are relevant in muscular development:

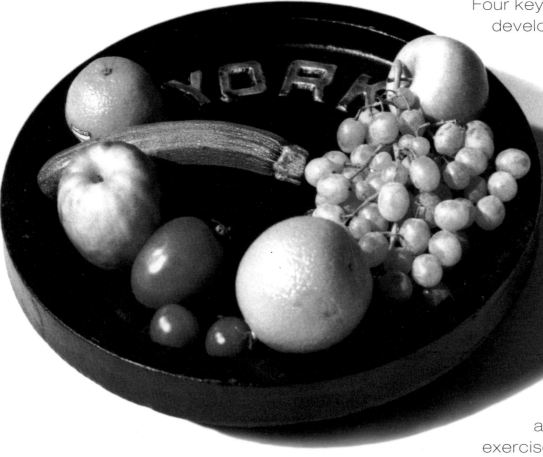

1 The quality – in terms of freshness, processing and composition – of the food you prepare and eat. Spending the amount of time you need to at the gym may make shopping for fresh ingredients difficult, but with the major supermarkets now staying open beyond work hours it is more practical than ever to shop for each meal you are about to prepare and eat.

2 The amount of food you eat. The more you eat, the more you grow, and provided any increase is balanced by exercise to burn the fuel created, your muscular strength and definition should increase accordingly. A larger appetite is the natural result of an increased physical activity, so it will be less like force feeding to achieve this increase in consumption than you would imagine.

3 The number and frequency of the meals you have. Research suggests that five or six smaller meals each day are better for you. Since eating causes a rise in the metabolic rate, five or six small meals will cause this to happen more often and so burn excess (fat) calories. For those unable to actually stop and take a formal meal at such regular intervals, nature has provided a handy fast food snack in the form of delicious fruits like apples and bananas, which can be eaten on the move, or at the desk. Canned or bottled protein drinks are much more widely available nowadays, and so can also be substituted for one or two of these light meals.

4 The content of your meals. Clearly, not all foods are as useful in a muscle development regime as others, and here follows a guide to help you plan for your main meals effectively. Sticking to it slavishly may seem boring, so have a day off now and again if you are finding yourself dissatisfied, though since this may lead to 'bingeing' it is a tendency best avoided.

A balanced meal features at least one item from each of the following groups:

Simple carbohydrate sources such as apples, pineapple, bananas, grapefruit, oranges, pears and grapes

Dairy (fat) sources such as low-fat milk, low-fat cottage cheese and non-fat yogurt

Protein sources such as chicken legs, lean beef, skinless chicken or turkey breast, fish, lamb or pork chops

Complex carbohydrate sources such as rice, pasta, potatoes and brown bread, pulses and beans, and all green vegetables

Opinion differs, but a guide for muscle building is a dietary ratio of 15% simple carbohydrates, 10% fat (but fat is present in all groups so you don't need so many actual fat sources), 30% protein and 45% complex carbohydrates will achieve a diet best for sustaining workouts and delaying the onset of fatigue.

In addition this meal content will also contain an ideal amount of fibre, the key factor in efficient food processing within the body.

PREMIUM FUELS

Even though healthy eating will undoubtedly help you achieve your goals, depriving yourself completely of any pleasures you may have enjoyed before your gym regime isn't compulsory. Remember to treat yourself – in moderation, and at the longest intervals you can manage – to your most missed favourites.

At all other times, try to eat as many of the high-nutrient foods described here. Fruit and vegetables should be as fresh as possible. Vegetables are best raw, but if boiled or steamed should be *al dente*. Meat should always be grilled.

Fruits The eminently portable snack food. **Bananas** are a rich source of potassium, thought to help regulate blood pressure, and provide fibre and act as a natural antacid into the bargain. **Figs** are in themselves quite messy to eat fresh, so a good snack and marvellous carbohydrate source – even during exercise sessions – are the fig bars you can get at health food shops and large supermarkets. **Dried fruit** is a good source of concentrated energy and iron (the latter helps prevent anaemia), and because it is high in fructose (natural sugars) can help satisfy a sweet tooth, but be fat-free. Apricots, pears, figs, raisins and bananas are the nicest. **Kiwi fruit** are useful little carbohydrate sources and are the gym-goer's picnic equivalent of a hard-boiled egg – take a teaspoon and scoop. **Papaya** has almost as rich a content of potassium as a banana, yet also contains nutrients galore. **Strawberries** are no longer limited to summer availability, and provide vitamin C and fibre in addition to a high proportion of carbohydrate.

Vegetables, pulses, pasta & grains

An excellent source of fibre, **beans** also provide protein and folic acid. Kidney, black and broad beans are best, but all beans are excellent. **Broccoli** is one of the most nutritious forms of food, providing fibre, vitamin C, folic acid, calcium, magnesium and iron, and has been linked to a reduced risk of various cancers. **Pasta** is good long-distance fuel, and is an excellent source of complex carbohydrates. There are also various types of enriched dried pastas to be found in health shops providing iron and vitamins. **Brown rice** is another great source of complex carbohydrates. It contains double the fibre of white rice and is an altogether richer fund of nutrients. **Corn** is a great source of fibre and carbohydrate, and has almost no fat, yet is often forgotten in the shopping basket. Fresh is nicest and best, but canned or frozen saves time. **Carrots** yield vitamin A and plenty of fibre, and cut into sticks are a great nibble for on the move. **Lentils** are a good source of protein and complex carbohydrates, and can act as an iron supplement. Unlike beans, they need no soaking and can be eaten on their own or added to soups. **Oatmeal** is a good source of soluble fibre, and in conjunction with a low-fat diet is frequently prescribed for lowering cholesterol levels. **Potatoes** are *the* basic fuel, and provide complex carbohydrates, and potassium. Remember that 'skin-on' will also ensure fibre is provided. **Wholegrain breakfast cereals** provide complex carbohydrates and fibre – but check that your chosen cereal has a low fat-to-fibre ratio.

Meat & fish If you are selective about its origins and careful to select lean cuts and trim excess fat, **beef** is still the great source of easily-absorbed iron, zinc and high-quality protein. **Chicken** without skin is now sold readily in the supermarket, and consequently contains very little fat, but plenty of iron and B vitamins. You can leave the skin on to stop the meat drying out during cooking, but be sure to discard it later. **Salmon** is a relatively low-fat, high protein food, and additionally yields special fatty acids and fish oils now widely judged to be beneficial. **Tuna** is the classic health and fitness food, and is the undisputed best staple of a high protein, low-fat diet. Fresh tuna, the most delicious form, is expensive and difficult to find, however. Tinned in brine is the best alternative.

Liquids A source of calcium and vitamin D, important for maintaining healthy bones, **skimmed milk** is low-fat, and an excellent base for liquidized fruit and vegetable shakes, which are another way of making snacks portable and convenient. **Fat-free yoghurt** is the healthy person's cream substitute, which is rich in vitamin B12 and calcium, and can be added to soups, casseroles, sauces, used for vegetable dips and to thicken liquidized drinks. Low-fat drinking yoghurts are now widely available too. Needed in the same way as a car needs oil to make it run, **water** is also the human engine's flushing system, and consequently needs constant topping-up. Unlike a car, it is not a sealed system: simple body cooling and bathroom trips lose you at least half a gallon daily, so once in an exercise regime you should never be without it. Drink a large glass about half an hour before exercising, and the same every 15 minutes during exercise. Most gyms provide water in a cooler these days, but you might want to think about taking a sports dispenser bottle with you to fill up and have with you so you don't forget to drink what is needed. As a miniumum throughout the day always drink a glass of water with each meal, and try to keep a glass to sip on your desk if you are at work. Your tank will be working its way towards empty just like the one in your car.

CARRYING CAPACITY

Eating sensibly is a bit of a struggle for even the most disciplined of us. Too often the battle that most people are trying to win is seen as the struggle between a **good** diet that emphasizes complex carbohydrates, and a **bad** diet featuring a heavy amount of fats. In reality your body needs both to survive, and a diet that is rich in carbohydrates and low in fat will be best.

Both fat and carbohydrates provide the body with fuel that is measured in calories. **Fat** contains about 9 calories per gram as opposed to carbohydrate's 4 calories per gram. Although fat contains more calories than carbohydrates, it is in reality how the body uses these calories that is important. Unless it has a need to, the body engine chooses not to burn fat as energy immediately, but causes it to be stored for later use. If you have a tendency to weight gain, and eat too much fat, you will quickly become overweight.

This storage facility is therefore a great nuisance to those trying to minimize body fat, but it provides at the same time a remarkable survival mechanism, since if you are unable to obtain food for a week or two it is this stored fat that the body draws on. Think of it as the 'reserve' tank that keeps you going after the low petrol warning light comes on.

This is the facility that allowed our ancestors to stalk their food for a couple of days without collapsing. Most of us have been lucky enough to avoid famine, and lead the sort of daily lives that are not routinely active, so do not require our 'reserve' tank at all. In spite of this we have not reduced our fat intake accordingly, and as a society actually consume more than our ancestors. Consequently, body fat is an issue.

To appreciate body fat control, you must understand how the body uses carbohydrates as fuel. Two types of carbohydrates exist: simple and complex. **Simple carbohydrates** are mainly found in fruits, and largely comprise natural sugars. The human digestive system turns them into blood sugar almost immediately they are consumed, providing instant fuel. This is the reason why a few dried apricots can provide a quick energy burst.

Obviously this type of energy boost could not suffice for all our needs. Not only is it fast-acting, but it is also fast-burning. The accelerator is on the floor, but the miles per gallon zooms down.

This is where **complex carbohydrates** come into play. They are the basic fuel in grains, pasta, bread, beans and other vegetables, and cannot be converted straight away into blood sugar. The chemistry is more complicated, so a slow and steady release of fuel into the bloodstream results. Eating complex carbohydrates is therefore the most sensible way of eating, since it lessens the need for simple carbohydrate top-ups and doesn't need you to draw on your fat reserves. Bad news, of course, if you are trying to lose some of that body fat.

The relationship between the various sources of calories is the key to shedding body fat. Your muscles consume blood sugar, or glycogen – their fuel – as you exercise. Glycogen is found in the muscles, the blood and the liver, and you draw on these three sources in that order, until they are all depleted.

Then one of two things happens. If you are exercising strenuously you will literally 'run out of fuel', and will be unable to continue without further fuel injection. If you sustain your exercise at a lower rate of exertion, however, the body will begin to draw on its fat reserves, and will do so during prolonged exercise periods even if the initial exercise were not very strenuous. Therefore, walking at a steady pace for a few hours burns more fat than an intensive run, simply because the run doesn't last long enough for the body to draw on the fat reserve.

In practice though, to lose body fat, exercise as intensely as you can, for as much time as you have available.

Controlling body fat by limiting your fat intake is a lot easier and healthier than trying to burn it off once it's with you. Simply replacing fats with complex carbohydrates is an effective way of losing weight without starving yourself.

FUEL INJECTION

Despite what you see on display in health food stores in the section for muscle-building, only one set of shelves in the store need interest you. A well-balanced and structured diet, a consistent gym plan and a healthy lifestyle with plenty of rest can be beneficially supplemented with vitamins and minerals taken in the form of pills and capsules. Most manufacturers provide literature explaining their products' virtues, but in simple terms there is no substitute for naturally present vitamins and minerals derived from a healthy diet. However, with modern food processing and chemically-controlled production methods, it is probably still important to 'top-up' your intake.

Unless you want to spend a great deal of money, and be unscrewing bottles for half an hour each day, a multi-vitamin and mineral combination may be the best solution for most of us. Brands are many and various, but all you really need to make sure of is that whatever you choose covers the vitamins and minerals listed in the table opposite.

You will not find a multi-vitamin that covers all the vitamin and mineral types in one pill, but be wary of the packaged 'one-day's worth' packets next to the till at the health food store, as they often represent bad value and contain things you don't want or need.

The fact that manufacturers do not seem to provide the one-pill wonder is not a question of marketing to get you to buy more than one product. A single pill with all the minerals and vitamins in in it would be literally rather hard to swallow.

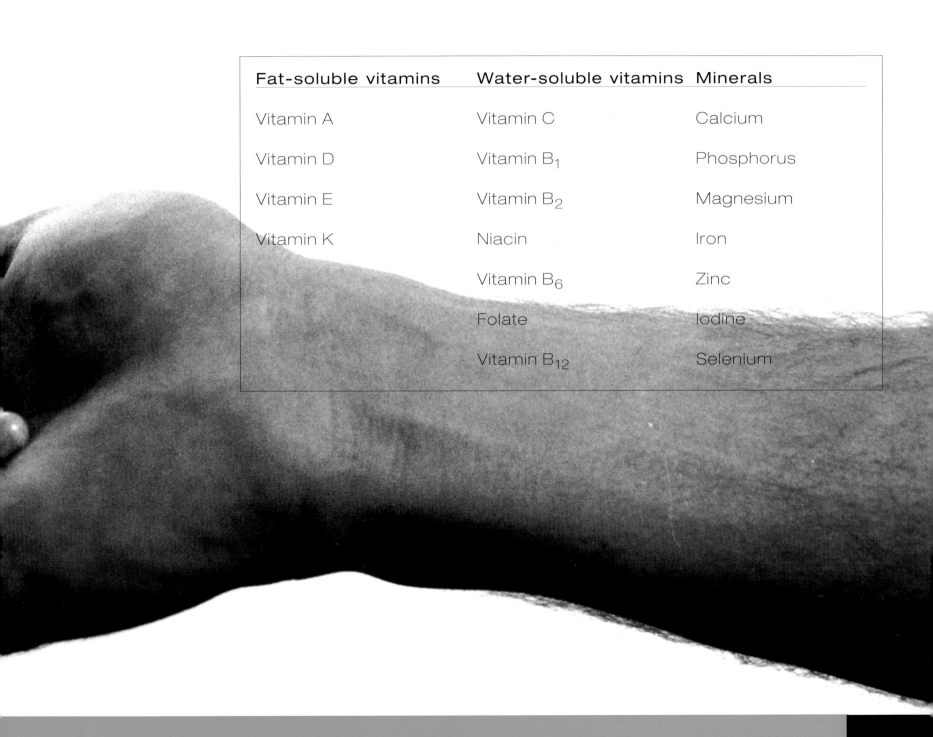

Fat-soluble vitamins	Water-soluble vitamins	Minerals
Vitamin A	Vitamin C	Calcium
Vitamin D	Vitamin B_1	Phosphorus
Vitamin E	Vitamin B_2	Magnesium
Vitamin K	Niacin	Iron
	Vitamin B_6	Zinc
	Folate	Iodine
	Vitamin B_{12}	Selenium

GLOSSARY

Arnold press A shoulder exercise involving the raising of a pair of dumb-bells vertically with a twisting motion.

Barbell A long bar with equal weights at each end.

Cable machine A machine incorporating a weight stack used in conjunction with a pulley, to which handles are attached. Two adjacent machines may be used together.

Cardio-vascular Exercise type designed to tax the heart muscles and increase blood flow.

Cool-down The process of lowering the body temperature after exercise.

Dumb-bell A short bar with equal weights at each end, supplied in pairs.

Exertion The positive 'weight moving' effort of any exercise movement (during which breath is exhaled).

Exhaustion The point at which no further complete repetition can be performed.

Fatigue Another term for the point at which no further complete repetition can be performed.

Free weights The term applied to non-machine gym weight training equipment, typically dumb-bells, fixed barbells, and bar and plates.

Isolation machine A gym machine designed to work one specific body part, usually with an adjustable weight stack.

Locking out The straightening out of a joint to its maximum.

Plate A round disc of varying weight, which can be loaded on to a bar, and held in place with a spring clip or screw collar.

Preacher The name applied to a special bench and exercise for which the arms are leant over a lectern-like pad.

Recovery The negative 'weight supporting' effort of any exercise movement (during which breath is inhaled).

Rep Short for repetition: the number of times an exercise can or should be performed.

Reverse flye machine A machine designed for back exercise, sitting facing the weight stack, but also used for chest exercise, by sitting facing away from the weight stack.

Set A number of reps, performed at the same time.

Smith machine The arrangement of a bar in a rack framework, at which certain exercises can be performed, with hook devices available to stop the bar and any loaded plates falling.

Stretch The process of stretching muscles out prior to, or following, strenuous exercise. May help prevent injury.

Weight stack An arrangement of rectangular weights in a pile, the quantity being selected by the use of a pin placed within the stack.

Z-bar A bar with a double zig-zag in it, used for arm exercises, and shorter than a straight bar.

Zottman curl An arm exercise involving rotational movements, designed to work the bicep.

All clothes by John Crummay, 43-45 Shorts Gardens, Covent Garden, London WC2, 0171 240 3534.

Photographed at Powerzone Health Club, 68-70 Putney High Street, London SW15, 0181 246 6700.

Black & white photographic printing and processing by Adrian Ensor, 0171 636 1739.

Senior Commissioning Editor for Boxtree/Pan Macmillan: Gordon Scott Wise.

Models: Sean Cochrane, John Walton, David Miller and Mark Miller at Boss Models, 0171 580 2444, and Dean Hodgkin.

Grooming: Fiona Corrigan and Maggie Hunt at Joy Goodman, 0181 968 6887.

The authors gratefully acknowledge the assistance of Ragdale Hall Health Hydro, 01664 434831.